WORD REMEDIES

A Collection

JANE O'SHEA

WILBUR PRESS
NEW ZEALAND

ISBN- 978-0-473-55799-7

Cover design by: Jess Le Marchand

www.wordremedies.co.nz

For Peter

PREFACE

Word Remedies help us to hear ourselves above the chatter and bustle of our daily lives. These words help to make sense of our messy inner landscapes, help to untangle the complexities of our relationships, and they reflect both our wonder at the world around us and our worry about what is happening to it.

With Word Remedies, we can begin unfamiliar and sometimes overdue conversations with ourselves and with others.

Word Remedies are soothing, provocative, and healing.

Table of Contents

INTRODUCTION

One day it happened. I couldn't wait any longer. Out of nowhere the thought hit me "you are halfway through your life and it's time to get on with it". I knew exactly what I was talking to myself about. Writing.

Realising that I couldn't hide from myself any longer, I rearranged my schedule so that I could have one morning a week to start doing the thing I'd been putting off for as long as I could remember. Thursday morning was it.

The first Thursday morning arrived with no distractions, no interruptions and to my great alarm, no words. With pen and paper, I first sat at my desk, then in my garden, then by the river, then tried walking through the forest – but nothing. By lunchtime I was agitated. Had this life-long dream to write been a delusion.

The next Thursday arrived and I pulled on my big-girl pants to give it another go. But by the end of morning, just like the first week, I had nothing but a few pages of crossed-out words. I was very unhappy and called myself a few choice words.

Deciding there had to be a better way, I called a writer friend and asked for help. He gave me two great pieces of writing advice.

First, to write only about what was important to me – what I felt, experienced, thought. So I starting writing about self-doubt and fear, and about the messiness of relationships. To write about what was right there, right then.

Second, he taught me to bear the first awful drafts, explaining that writing was a big messy word-vomit followed by editing, editing, editing.

So the next Thursday I had a huge word vomit – pages and pages of it. This gave me enough material to edit away for many Thursdays to come.

Somewhere along the way I have learnt to endure all the bad writing that comes out of me. I've also learnt to discipline myself to edit for as long as it takes, and to be unafraid of discarding something no matter how long I have worked on it.

That was 2003. As you will see, I have distracted myself over and over since I started this writing lark 18 years ago.

This book is a collection of 259 word remedies. 85 are included in my first book *Follow Yourself Home,* 110 are in my second book *In Your Smallest Pocket,* and the last 64 haven't been published before.

I have written about what has meaning for me, and what I have observed in others. Writing is my most challenging, and at the same time, most rewarding endeavour. The plan is to keep writing for the rest of my life as there are still a few books up my sleeve. Though judging from past experience, I'm sure to wobble off course from time to time.

Writing this book has been remedial for me. I hope that reading it will be the same for you.

STARTING

January 2003 - February 2004

A TIME WHEN

Words and phrases keep popping into my head, reminding me that I have always wanted to be a writer. I realise that I'm half way through my life and it's time to get on with it. All those things I would do someday … that day was now.

I'd given a copy of my very first poem to a friend and noticed it stuck on his fridge. He tells me that he reads it often and it helps. I'm dumbfounded. Maybe I can do this, maybe it's time to give it a serious go. Maybe.

THAT SOLID PLACE

I am no longer content
to let anyone else's opinion of me
mean more than my opinion of myself

I am no longer content
to give up my own true
wants, needs, thoughts and opinions
because someone else
believes something different

I am no longer content
to let my mind get caught in those old traps
that take me to that old place
that does me no good

To go there
leaves me collapsed
leaves me lost
leaves me confused
leaves me exhausted

I own and treasure that solid place inside of me
and nurture it and cradle it
and won't give it up
for any reason
at any time
for anyone

It is mine and I need this
more than I need anything else
more than I need love
more than I need acceptance
more than I need validation

I need me to believe in me

January 2003 (1)

THE STILL SILENT TREES

All you need do is breathe out
and everything else takes care of itself

With each breath
the air, christened by the silent trees
enters you warmed and loved
then is released into a waiting world

From your first breath at birth
rhythmed and measured
until the last breath of your surrender
And each breath in between
announcing your blessed place

Breath after breath
connecting you to everything
in this lively sea of air

February 2003 (2)

ON OUR KNEES

Marriage is sacred
Not because it is sanctified by God
but because it brings us to our knees

Kneeling on the cold wooden floor
we are asking for blessings
we are asking for answers
How to love
How to be loved

A yearning heart
sitting before the altar of love
candles lit in worship

A screaming heart
standing before the vast despair
arms raised, raging

A silent heart
kneeling before itself
eyes closed in hope

All asking
How to love
How to be loved

March 2003 (3)

THE WHOLE OF MY LIFE

For the whole of my life
I have hidden myself
believing that I am not good enough

For the whole of my life
I have stood behind someone else
complaining they are in my way

For the whole of my life
I have denied my creative spirit
by spending my time
doing every thing else

Now, I can stand on the mountain of my life
and appreciate all that I am
Now, I walk beside the seemingly infinite ocean
and watch as the river empties
itself into that great expanse
Embracing the creative emptiness within me

And now
I honour my creative spirit
to breathe
to create
and to celebrate

July 2003 (4)

A DIVINE SWEETNESS

I woke this morning
to a divine sweetness
in my mouth

In the night
someone had forgiven me

Or perhaps it was I
who had forgiven

July 2003 (5)

THE MARRIAGE VOWS

I will hurt you, this I can promise
for if I don't, then this is not love

I want you rough and raw
not some smooth and shiny version
that may suit me better
And I will not always change for you
We will not always fit
This I can promise

Sometimes when you come to me small and fragile
I will fail you
This too I can promise
Forgive me

You will know my fury
You will know my withdrawal
I will blame you
This I can promise
Again - forgive me

In the sometimes conflict and confusion
I will not dull myself
so we can live in numbed compliance
I promise to stay present and alive with you

And yes, there will be love and lust, laughter and joy
that's the easy part

You will not be everything I want
and I promise to still want you
When I see you lacking
I promise to look away

And each morning
I promise to come back to you
my body and my heart open

This is my offering to you
These are my vows

January 2004 (6)

THE FENCE BY MY HEART

Love followed me home once
and sat on my fence
watching

Love sat patiently
waiting for me to finish my chores
and notice

Love, sitting on the fence by my heart
got tired and wandered off

Now Love only visits
every second Sunday and on Public Holidays

Still sits on the fence by my heart
waiting for me to notice

January 2004 (7)

A TREE'S LAMENT

They began to fall, my beautifully admired flowers
Such agony to see them turn to rags
But still I had my glorious leaves
shiny and green and silver in the summer breeze
Proudly giving shelter and beauty

As the nights became colder and the days shorter
I was terrified as my adorning leaves
turned yellow and red and brown
and began to fall
The earth, however
was happy to wear my handsome colours

Shy and raw, I was stripped of my handsome attire
and it would not stop, not until I was naked
With no admiring eyes to feast on me
I was alone through the long winter stillness

I decided to be a perfect tree
My twigs and branches would not litter the ground
I'd drink up all the best nutrients
and grow straight and tall with the most fragrant flowers
If I was good, all would be well again

Then, unannounced, my sap started to rise
Life entered me and growth began
Bursting soft shoots of green and gold
and the birth to a myriad of festive flowers

All spring and summer I was happy
useful and beautiful
A good tree
Then it happened again
my flowers and leaves deserted me
My humiliation was bared for all to see

Angry
I threw my branches in the strong winds
intent on destruction
I grew at annoying angles and rebelled
against the nature that tortured me
And still it happened, over and over
tedious in its repetition
I could not enjoy the delights of spring and summer
for fear of winter and autumn

Until at last, slowly, slowly, slowly, I learnt
To savour the still quiet of my winter's rest
To appreciate the colourful promise of spring
Celebrate the frivolous joys of my summer
And accept the inevitable letting go of autumn

January 2004 (8)

HERE AT LAST

And I finally showed up in my life
And it's halfway through
And that's how long it takes

To give back everything
everything that is not mine

Relieved
at last
I am here

At the centre of my own life
At the centre of my own life

January 2004 (9)

BREATHING SPACE

It does not matter
if I please you
or if you look at me with loving eyes
None of this matters
to the queen of my own heart

What matters
is that I smile inwardly
at my own failings
forgiving
And open each day to my own goodness

That I soothe and soften my own wandering mind
and give space to my own thoughts and dreams

That I breath long and slow into my soft belly
and I know my own song by heart

January 2004 (10)

THIS WAS NOT THE PLAN

We are the baby boomers
We went to Woodstock
We weren't supposed to get old

Bulging bellies
skin that no longer fits
hair growing in all the wrong places

I am a baby boomer
I believed in the sixties
I'm not supposed to get old

And by the way
Who stole my libido
Who changed the plan

February 2004 (11)

THIS GLORIOUS DAY

Daylight prises open my eyelids
nudging me into this glorious morning

The sun is bemused that I do not
leap from sleep
grab hold of the day
and shake it upside down
for all the treasure it holds

Fear stops me from gathering to my heart
all that is good and true and solid
Scared that if I truly let it in
it could be taken away and then I might
break into pieces beyond repair

This gift
so abundantly given
I keep at a distance for fear of loss
And so I do lose
a little of life every day

February 2004 (12)

LONG PATIENT TIME

You don't know me
You fell over me one night and decided to stay

You see me as means to your salvation
redemption in the soft folds of my body
It is a dream, a myth
to believe we can find a saviour
to make it all better
to make each other all better

To see each other, really see
To forgive ourselves and each other
To know, really know each other

Takes time
unholy time
unravelling time
long patient time

February 2004 (13)

JUST TESTING

I will test you
you who dares to love me

Three tasks to prove to me
that you are true
Ah, but not so easy
as the tasks of old
To slay the dragon
steal the troll's tooth
and the key from under the witch's pillow

For you, who dares to love me
much greater feats are asked

That you have me receive your gifts of love
so I believe myself worthy of such riches

That you have me trust that you will stay
and vanquish my fear that you will abandon me

That you have me deeply feel my need for you
so I reclaim the softness of my own fragile heart

These three tasks I set for you, my love
And then I may, perhaps
say yes

And after the yes
from time to time
I will test you again
Just to make sure
Just in case

February 2004 (14)

HOLDING HANDS

All you ever need do is hold my hand
you don't have to carry me

When I fall
I need to find my own way up
All you need do is lend me your reassuring hand

When I have rubbed myself raw, struggling against life
I just need the gift of your soothing hand to hold
while I find my way through

And when I am wild with passionate blame
convinced you are wrong
don't fight me or leave me
Sit with me and hold my hand

When I am tired
take my hand and show me to my bed

When I am confused, you don't need to fix me
I need to recognise my own knowing

When I believe myself broken and ask you to carry me
refuse, and offer me your loving hand
I will remember my wholeness

I need to feel my feet on this solid earth
All you ever, ever need do
is walk with me and simply hold my hand

February 2004 (15)

BELIEVING

March 2004 - November 2004

A TIME WHEN

I get braver and start to take writing more seriously, though still squeezing it in-between running my business and attending to my family. I start doing a few performances and I make a CD. I establish a mercurial relationship with writing - sometimes flowing freely, other times strangled by doubt. I have, however, found that deeply satisfying creative place inside me and long to take up residence.

THE VOICE CALLING YOU HOME

Take off your muddied work coat
toiling so hard to make yourself something else
Stop shouting for your work to finish
you need simply to open the door

Open the door and come right in
You will find the handle
on the inside of your heart
Someone has left the light on
with a note to welcome you home

Someone will serve you
a rich moist pudding
the time for celebration has come
Time for you to stop my friend
your searching has come to an end

Take off your dusty traveller's boots
leave them right there on the road
Someone has run you a long hot bath
you can soak as long as you please

Leave your taskmaster's clothes on the doorstep
as someone has laid out your artist's clothes
They are clean and bright
smelling expectant and new
waiting patiently here for you

Someone has turned back and warmed your bed
fragrant pillows to welcome you in
and an old familiar voice hums to you soft and low

Saying
It's time for you to come home and rest
It's time to come in from the cold

March 2004 (16)

THE FEAST

All these years
I have been hungry
Lying in dream next to you as we sleep
All this time, starving myself
when you have been right here at my table

To move beyond my need for you
to feel my greed
I want to feast on you
every last morsel
Eat of you until I cannot move
I groan and I ache
I am so full of you

No elegant tea party for me
I want to dig in with both hands
eat with my fingers
The juices run down my arms
and over my rolled-up sleeves
I'll slurp, and I'll most heartily burp
as I devour this banquet of you

You need not excuse me
for I will not apologise
Table manners be damned
I have waited long enough

The smell of your freshly showered body
crisp and crunchy, ripe for the picking
enticing me to take a bite
Your toasted toes
Your buttocks, risen to perfection
Each ounce of you a delight

Dark rich chocolate of your eyes
you're a sweet and luscious dessert, my love
I'll lick the bowl clean, every last taste
with my sticky fingers
I will partake of you

Roasted, my fattened lamb
I'll carve succulent slices of you as you sleep
A midnight feast
My gluttony knows no bounds

I drink to you, my love
the deep red wine running down my chin
over my shirt, staining my skin

And I will sleep replete each night, divinely drunk
divinely drunk, intoxicated with you
and wake each morning once more
to my hunger and to my greed

March 2004 (17)

THE CUPBOARD IS EMPTY

I can't take care of you anymore
I'm tired, I'm spent
The well is dry
the cupboard empty
It's time for me to shut up shop

I know you are hungry
that you are thirsty
in need of nourishment
But then, so am I
If you ask me again
you will find me cold and closed

I must go and find my own golden fields to harvest
my own spring water to drink

And if you do the same
then maybe we can share supper again
and drink from the same cup once more

March 2004 (18)

HOLDING MYSELF AGAINST THE WORLD

Sitting here
holding my breath against the world
Resentful that life isn't serving me
hot tea in bed each morning
Pulling back because love isn't
given in a nice neat package each Christmas

Here I am pulling back
holding in, screwing up my eyes
Pretending that I do not want
that I do not need

Perhaps
I can dare to dream it
That thing that is almost too painful to imagine
I can stay brave
even when life hits me hard
even when it aches a hole right through me

Keep my hands outstretched
my eyes wide open
my breath soft and easy
and keep asking

And my life will ripen
a most bountiful crop

March 2004 (19)

ODE TO A COMPETENT WOMAN

You can do everything
but why would you want to
Just because you can do something
doesn't mean you have to

What you possibly do need
is a good dose of incompetence

March 2004 (20)

MY OWN DELICATE HEAD

Sanity hits me full in the face
when at last I notice
that the madness I listen to
comes from inside my own head

Such a small space
So full of judgement, argument, complaint
and imagined injustice
I have lists and shoulds and won't s and shouldn'ts
to dos and to don'ts
he said, she said, they didn't, why won't
I'll never, when will, why me
I can't and on and on
you always, you never, my turn, you said, I want, I need
and on and on and on and on and on

Sometimes a dull drone in the background
Often a cacophony of noise
drowning out any possibility of an original thought
All inside my own delicate head
and often pouring out my mouth – eyh

Don't believe everything that goes on
inside my head

It's madness
Mostly madness

March 2004 (21)

LOST CHILD

In the river flow of my life
sometimes I drift into the black waters along the banks
Stuck between the green-grey stones
Stagnant
The tiny hovering insects
dead leaves and twigs, stale and lifeless

Shadows move
and the lost and lonely abused child
crawls from deep within me once more

She appears in different forms

Sometimes small and tight
and I cannot breathe
Sometimes huge and horrible
and I shake and cannot move
Sometimes empty and alone
and I cannot feel anything - numb
Sometimes she screams and rages
and I frighten the hell out of myself
Sometimes she is sad and young
and I rock her back to sleep
Sometimes stoic and hard
and I beat myself with it
Sometimes fragile and she cracks
and I don't know what to do
Sometimes it's tedious, just plain tedious
and I want it to go away
Sometimes she cries tears of shame and loss
and I sigh with relief
Sometimes she lies to me
and I'm mean and call myself names
Sometimes she pushes me hard
pushes me to accept, to forgive and to change

But mostly she sleeps, quiet and content
in the still shadows and dark waters within me
Life flows and the river moves me on
and all is well

Sometimes, the past superimposes on the present
and the wounded child returns
showing the scars indelibly made so long ago
The wounds have healed, the scars remain
always part of everything

I do not understand why
All I know is that for some unfathomable reason
I need to go deep within to that child
To hold and to cradle
To sing and to soothe
To listen and reassure

To wade in and pull her out of the black water
the moving shadows
and reassure her on her way

I am that child and I am her guardian

And the river flows again
The river always flows again

March 2004 (22)

I'LL SEE YOU TOMORROW

Wake carefully, slowly
staying deep inside
Any rogue thoughts
are asked to come back tomorrow
Tomorrow I will go visiting the world

Today I stay home
Today I go wandering inside my own inner landscapes
Today I meet with myself

Go for a walk with my dreams
stretch their legs
Settle back in a big soft cushion
watch my imaginings on the big screen
Hot chocolate with my fears
giving them a reassuring hug
Pack up my self-doubts and send them off on holiday
they have been working overtime for far too long

Tomorrow I will answer the telephone
pay the mortgage
feed the kids

Today I wake gently
greeting myself with big welcoming arms

Today I'll see myself
I'll see you tomorrow

March 2004 (23)

CONFESSION

We are careless with our words
They can sting and singe the fragile hearts
of those we meet and those we love
Each unkind word a poison arrow

Then we wonder why some hearts harden
why eyes turn away, why people separate

But it's not as simple as catching the words
before they escape
The judgements we hold in our thoughts
are prisons that isolate
Each unkind word an iron bar across our heart
We become caught in barbed wire
not knowing how to free ourselves

Time to call back each unkind word and thought
Invite them home like wayward youth
so we can know them
wrestle with them, listen and forgive

Own them as we would our own children
to find counsel and acceptance within us

March 2004 (24)

LOVE ME THE MOST

Love me the most
when I deserve it the least

Feed me sweetness
when my mouth is bitter

Massage my hard heart
when I close

It is not you I fight with
It is myself

March 2004 (25)

MOST WILDLY BEAST

My life, a wildly beast
a most wildly beast
Hurtling off in every direction as
I hold fiercely to his tail
Gripping tight, as the beast rushes through
my hectic world
I'm flung and thrown, this way and that
reacting to all the things I bang into
Feeling more and more giddy and bruised

Too scared to let go
Panicked
that my wildly beast will run away without me
Too busy complaining that I'm too busy
too important, too tired, too indispensable
Too busy being stoic and heroic to notice
that all I need do is let go

And let go I surely do - finally
And my wildly beast does come wandering back
wondering where I am
most apologetic
and asks me to climb back on his back
Riding high on it's shoulders
We're galloping off again

And then I forget
as life urgently demands
that I attend to the world

And surely
I only look away for just a moment
and the slide begins
as I slowly slip down his furry back

Too busy attending to other things to notice
and before I know it
I'm clutching his tail
tossed about
wondering

How did I get here again

April 2004 (26)

AOTEAROA

She rose from of her mother's molten core
born through a salty embryonic fluid
into a great birthing sea

Lapping waves nursed her body
long winds kissed her flushed cheeks
wandering rivers quenched her parched lips
Ecstatic birdsong proclaiming her arrival
here in these southern oceans
far away from the conforming crowds

Down here with space to grow her wild heart
she formed her fearless mountains
With reverence she planted her trees and ferns
With innocence her beauty overflowed
and with generosity she welcomed all her people

I am in love with this land
deeply honoured to belong to these people
On these sacred islands I claim my place

Enthralled and enchanted as I watch us grow
Sometimes shy and self-conscious
daring and brave

Standing here before a curious world

April 2004 (27)

THE QUIET CURVE OF SURRENDER

For so long I would not trust in a life that let babies die
that poisoned our hearts so that we could hurt and kill
A life where forests burn and families separate

And so I remained self-righteous and aloof
in my scepticism and condemnation
Orphaned by my own cynicism and doubt

I still do not know why babies need to die
I do know however, that I want to ride
the agonising edge of faith

To relinquish the need for life to follow my rules
To welcome the drama
the complexity, the foolishness
the contradiction, the paradox
the conflict, the futility
the illogical, the absurd
the senseless and the disgrace

To concede to the mystery
To know it is unknowable
To rest my cheek
on the quiet curve of surrender

May 2004 (28)

MY CHILD LEAVES HOME

You tumbled into my heart
I fell hopelessly in love with you
from the first time I spied your tiny eyes
Awe and terror that something so precious
that smelled so pure
could be given into my care

I long to know that I have done good enough

I wanted so much to do it perfectly
to mother you as I was never mothered
give you the life I had always dreamed
But real life and my humanness got in the way
If I find fault, it is not criticism of you
but my own guilt at my own failings

That I could save you from the fire of your own life
that my struggle could take away yours
and my suffering could protect you from pain

All I can do is admire you
admire you into your life
Rejoice in you, everything
Watch breath-taken as you create your world

Forgive me for my mistakes
Honour me for doing the best that I could
Share with me all the worlds you find
and come back to me
in the spaces between

May 2004 (29)

THIS UNHOLY MADNESS

The heart is chaotic
Our inner world comic in its contradictions and jumble
Yet we measure ourselves daily
against the reality of life's disarray
Coming up wanting in our need for order and sense

We order our lives with schedules and lists
rules neatly piled and filed
in the hope that such tidiness
will seep through our skin
and our insides will stay neatly folded

Ah, that when we were made
all of us would make sense
That we could understand
the complex maze of our humanness
And present ourselves designed with
reason and logic, rational and suitable
with everything sorted and civilised

We turn from the sight of our struggles
as we dull ourselves so our madness will not show

Instead
Let us celebrate our madness
let it go rampant
Let's experience this living drama
unfettered, unrehearsed, raw and tender
Let's explore our messy cupboards
where all the treasure and jewels are hidden

Then we can sit together unafraid
Judgements aside
let's revel in the irreverent truth

Revealing ourselves to each other
surprised as we discover
the depths and degrees
of this unholy madness

May 2004 (30)

THE EMPTY HAND OF DOUBT

Self doubt lives in the very marrow of my bones
infiltrating my blood
pulsing through my body
The slightest graze and out it oozes

Doubt sits between my breaths
behind my thoughts
Filling all the spaces that should be left
for dreaming and scheming
Irritating the soft tissue of my imagination

Doubt is tricky, uses many names
and always has excuses
Masquerades with cunning disguises
Doubt loves to procrastinate

Doubt wants me to
trip over myself
So I don't make any mistakes
and stay secure in my small safe world

When I go to find myself
instead I find the empty hand of doubt
I am defeated before I start
and never know the relief
when self doubt
finally leaves me alone

June 2004 (31)

WITHOUT QUESTION

The day is over

I sit here in wonder
as the tide inches in
The cooling sea moving over my feet
touching the salted sweat on my skin
Reminding me of my briny beginnings

With all the devastation and neglect
she still faithfully wakes us each morning
To give without question
all that she has

Each morning and each night
the earth turns and bows
her great oceans moving
over her generous body
and the water moves over
my grateful feet

June 2004 (32)

LOVE ONLY LIVES IN WIDE OPEN SPACES

I withdraw my love
punishment for your hurting
my delicate heart
Hiding away in a vain attempt
to keep out the hurt

Bruised and alone
I withdraw even further
into the lost wilds of my inner protection
Caught in an elaborate maze
to protect my vulnerable heart

As I look out from these barred windows
all seems deserted and withheld
All my carefully laid plans
my clever escape routes
They have failed
for still I hurt

Because love only lives in wide open spaces
only thrives in vast expansive places

Time to dismantle the barricades
and open the door
peep around the corner
and venture outside

July 2004 (33)

FOLLOW YOURSELF HOME

Following life as it demands that you venture
further and further out into the world
Until you become caught in your own forgetting
and find yourself far away from where your dreams began
Promising you will take care of yourself soon

At last, stopping
bewildered and dazed
The enchanted forest has become bleak and black
and you are lost
too long away from your heart's home

Time to leave the responsibilities still asking
and the tasks unfinished
Close your ears to the screaming complaints
and the unending demands

Hold still and listen
to the faint and distant rhythm that is your own
and follow and follow and follow
Until you recognise yourself in your step
and follow and follow and follow
Until you remember
and know yourself once more
Until you settle back into your own relieved body
and vow to never get lost again

That with each adventure out into the world
you will always come home to yourself
and rest

July 2004 (34)

COMING OUT OF HIDING

I am tired of playing love's hide-and-seek with you
My heart goes stale waiting for you to find me

I want to stand before you unashamed
look into your eyes
and ask for what I need

And listen to you with clear and undefended ears

I want to live with you honestly
and lay with you unafraid

I may fail you
I may trip over myself

But I will not hide from you anymore

July 2004 (35)

AS EASY AS THE DAY MOVES

Life piled up on top of me
body aching under the strain
Mind stoic, pushing on
Breath gripping, intense and tight
Eyes fixed and unseeing
Heart forgotten

I'm tired and undone

To live as easy as the day moves
always trusting in the coming of night
Separate my compacted thoughts
and move into the precious spaces inside my body
Untie my heart threads
to find love's loose and open weave
Soften my eyes so I can
look again with compassion and relief

To live as easy as the day moves
easy as the draping of night
easy as dawn's silent light easing into the day
easy as breathing in and breathing out
breath received and breath surrendered

As easy as opening my eyes

July 2004 (36)

THE STORIES WE TELL

The stories we tell ourselves
The stories we tell
That old tattered book
with those old tired stories
Told so many times
We're almost convinced they're true

Blindly living out our stories
as if they are real
Steadfastly believing every line
every pause, every word

We define ourselves
by these worn-out stories
Tall tales of woe and want
heartbreak and betrayal
Rigid stories with tedious plots
goodies and baddies
solid full-stops and
devoid of any question marks

Then your story and mine collide
and the battle begins
To prove the validity of my story
and the delusion of yours

Turn the page, shut the book
throw away the bookcase, the lot

Greet each day with an adventurous pen in hand
ready to write this new day's story

September 2004 (37)

MY HORMONES ANSWERED THE DOOR

Woke up, got out of bed
fell off my perch head first into the shit

My hormones proceeded to answer the door
and everything that walked through
after that was wrong

Someone, believing they were talking to me
inadvertently addressed my hormones
who answered without logic or sense

Wading through this sea of oestrogen
I finally found my old friend chocolate
who sat with me and helped me feel better

By evening my hormones and I
had come to an understanding

Now
I know my hormones may be useful
but I wish they wouldn't cause such havoc
in an otherwise peaceful life

October 2004 (38)

TUMBLING PAST OUR DOOR

Life is supposed to be a mystery
not a foregone conclusion
We pay our dues
for the experience
not for the set of plans

It's not an endurance test, a race, a destination
or even an exam we need to get right
It is a strange and mystifying adventure

A pilgrimage
to find the way to our sacred heart
To find we are already right here at home

So we can know the divine and the ordinary
in each and every moment and movement of life
as it tumbles past our door

Give up the struggle
for life already knows
what it is doing

November 2004 (39)

FIND ME

You knocked on my door
I didn't invite you
You asked to come in

But my heart decided long ago
to never be hurt like that again
So I turned the key tightly
and turned you away

There is no key to my heart
I just pretend that it is locked away

My heart weeps from its far away place
desperately hoping
that you will find me

November 2004 (40)

GETTING SERIOUS

January 2005 - December 2005

A TIME WHEN

I take my notebook everywhere with me, still fitting writing around everything else. I wake early and write every day. I write in the supermarket carpark. I write going for long walks up the river valley. I write while waiting for the kids outside school. I truly believe I'm on my way and it feels like I will never stop. Little do I know.

IN DENIAL

My need wanders about
listless and lonely in its denial
Not knowing what to do with itself

My need
a dog desperately searching for attention
My need
a scurrying mouse
hiding, always hiding
My need
a cat slinking around looking
for the most comfortable lap to plunder

My need denied
gets up when I do
and follows me about

I need you to respond to me
smile in recognition
answer in response
receive with gratitude
know me in my struggle
see me in my glory
forgive me in my ignorance
honour me in my triumph

And I need you to need me
so I can feel my relevance
in connection to you

January 2005 (41)

THE ONLY ROAD HOME

Did I leave this day unlived
Did I wander off

Finding myself in a deluge of doubt
veering off into fear, lost in the future

Or slipping below the surface
sinking into the past
drowning in resentment or regret

Neither doubt nor resentment live in the present
They are thieves that rob me of now
this moment
the only place I can truly live

Forgiveness
the only path back from the past

Trust
the only road home

January 2005 (42)

IN YOUR SMALLEST POCKET

You wake each day
to this bewildering world
and again wonder
What am I doing

Your life, eaten away
diced and sliced
into meaningless portions
Served up to the God of lists
and things yet to be done

In the smallest pocket
of your oldest clothes
you will find it
Right where you left it
in your busyness and inattention

It doesn't matter how much harder you try
in your discontent and longing
For there, in your smallest pocket
your happiness is waiting still

All you need do is remember
Smile to yourself at your forgetfulness
slide in your hand
hold tight
And there you will find it
your happiness waiting still

February 2005 (43)

GETTING OVER MYSELF

No more dragging my heavy heart stone
out of bed each morning
Trudging through a sticky quagmire
of bitter resentment
Hauling and heaving my great boulders of blame

Time to get over myself

Even through the agony of forgiveness
Even through the screaming voices demanding
that I hold on to my rightness
Even through the fear that I will lose
Even through the injustice of it not being fair

It is time

February 2005 (44)

FINALLY SHE KNEW

She searched and she searched
but she could not find God

Buddha's temple, Christ's church
Mohammad's mosque, Krishna's garden
They all left a fragrant trail
that kept her searching and searching
But still she could not find God

She looked within
finding a myriad of intriguing things
Kept her amused for years
And still God eluded her

She read the books
listened to the great masters' words
She prayed
Still nothing
Failure haunted her in her search for the Divine
Could so many find God but not her

Finally she stopped
She was still
And she found it
It was right there beside her, singing
celebrating with her in laughter
loving her through her children's eyes
lying with her as she bathed
feasting with her at her table

And finally she knew

February 2005 (45)

CURL-UP-IN-BED LOVE

To make the other wrong when they are hurting
just leaves them harsh or distant
They react
and we descend down
the steep slide of resentment

We can see the hurt
but we cannot always help
We can understand
but it's hard to make it better

When their hurt turns them into
someone we do not like
All we can do is love them
A soft, fragile, light-as-butterfly love
and wrap them up and take the world away
Not jump-in-the-deep-end love
but quiet-soothing love
Not wide-open-spaces love
but curl-up-in-bed love

And us too
when we are unlovely
we need indulgent, forgiving love
Just for a while
until our bruises lose their colour
and our wounded heart can lift its head
to see past the hurt

March 2005 (46)

DIRTY DISGUSTING BAD HABIT

Just when I think the divorce papers have been settled
Bad Habit creeps in the side door
and steals into my bed
I turn over and there he is caressing me with his sly words
"It's me you love, you know it's me you love"
Seducing me with his treacherous words
promising to make it all better

So hard to resist
my old lover Bad Habit
So very hard to resist
You'd think I'd see through him by now
I've fallen for his cunning tricks so many times before
You'd think I'd have learnt by now

Oh no
Bad Habit invites himself for late night supper
then hides in my fridge
calls to me from the pantry
"It's me you love, you know it's me you love"

He loses my walking shoes
reorganises my diary
convincing me to do it his way

So I almost forget what I really want
Lying and underhanded
he turns up in so many places
Always unhelpful
Dirty disgusting Bad Habit

March 2005 (47)

THE PRECISE MOMENT OF CHOICE

It is not the job I do
the size of my house
who I love or what I say
that makes up the total of how I live
It is each small habit
Those choices I make each minute
that sculpt my life

A better life doesn't come from wishing or wanting
complaining or resenting
from therapy or pushing or trying harder
But from the still moments between
a thought and its action
The precise moment when I can choose

Not the habitual life I have settled for
or the conditioned life I have inherited
or the hurried life I have manufactured
or even the fantasy life I may have imagined

No blinding flash of enlightenment
but the mindful life I choose
when I breathe out
before I breathe in

To notice these spaces
between impulse and action
between thought and deed
is to choose consciously how I live

April 2005 (48)

AND I STAND HERE NOW

From the time this planet began
hurtling through space
and the sun caught her in its orbit

From the first moment when life began from nothing
the smallest idea, the tiniest spark
and each fragment of growth
From that time, eons upon eons
many miracles happened
And I stand here now

That each ancestor, from the tiniest to now
multiplied, replicated, to evolve, to develop
always finding a way to reproduce
to grow and mature
And I stand here now

Each living thing that found nourishment
each meal to stay alive
And I stand here now

Through millions of years
during vast change and huge challenge
stories of courage, endurance and determination
the driving force to continue
And I stand here now

All the failures that fell away
mistakes that led to nowhere
and still enough survived
And I stand here now

And sight and taste and touch
and smell and sound and speech
and then love and art
thought and heroism and beauty
compassion, philosophy and joy

And I stand here now

Humbled at the persistence
in awe of the patience
grateful for the success
overwhelmed at the magnitude

And I stand here now

April 2005 (49)

WRAP ME UP WARM

Adorn me with your smile
I will become more beautiful

Praise me with your tender words
I will glow in gratitude

Anoint me with your kindness
I will grow more trusting

Feed me with your loving touch
a full belly is what I need

And kiss me and kiss me and kiss me

Wrap me up warm in your acceptance
watch me melt away

Spoil me until I am impossible
Spoil me with your opened heart

Indulge me
my beloved
Indulge me
with love

May 2005 (50)

MENDING MY MIND

Worrying makes holes in my head
and the good bits keep falling out
Then the wind blows
my thoughts into disarray

The more I anxiously scramble
to keep my thoughts in order
the more my brain leaks
The goodness, leached and lost

I want to mend my mind
Plug up the holes
with trust and resolve
Then my mind can find solutions
my fretting-thoughts could never find

And I might even think of something
I hadn't thought of before

May 2005 (51)

A LIFE-GIVING KISS

Each moment
a delicate life-giving kiss
Life choosing me again

In just a blink
my eyes are presented
with detailed beauty

Such exquisite touch
caressing, holding, belonging

Sound connecting
delighting, soothing

My heart is satisfied
with love so constant
it remains no matter how much
I give or deny

What can I give in return
What can I give
but gracious gratitude

June 2005 (52)

WAGING WAR WITH OUR DEMONS

Everyone has a great battle
the fight
that hard thing that takes us
again and again into the drama

We all have a great battle
with lack of stability, lack of money
with depression, addiction, shame or pain
confusion, loss, disability, illness
fear or doubt or shyness
lack of nurturing and love
We know our own inner conflict

Yet we shamefully hide our struggles
each of us left feeling alone in our dramas
Fearing exposure, we hide
believing in our own unique flaw

Everyone has a great battle
whatever they would lead you
to see or believe
So have compassion for your own

And when you see another's struggle
judgements aside, look with soft and kind eyes
remembering that somewhere in our lives
we are waging war with our own demons

Life is not wrong because we battle
life is made good through our battles
We are not broken because we struggle
we are made whole through our struggles

June 2005 (53)

DANCING THROUGH YOUR GARDEN

It's gratitude that keeps
the heart strong
That melts the fear
and breaks the spell

It's gratitude that opens the door
and shows the way
That answers the questions
that worry the mind
and close the heart

It's gratitude that has
a thousand happy pixies
dancing through your garden
Throwing blessings
sowing seeds of grace
upon your life

June 2005 (54)

THE ARGUMENT

We lost our way somewhere
between our head and our heart

Waylaid by our words
justifying ourselves
convincing each other
Arguing streams of freezing words

Until all we have gained
is an insurmountable mountain of words
Until we hit the chilling heights of silence
and a glacier slowly carves
a widening chasm between us

Our hearts harden under the weight
Painful echoes clog the cool air
All passes closed

Then the tiniest crack
Just the smallest crevice of hope

July 2005 (55)

THAT GOD COULD BE SO CLUMSY

God breaks me open, again
I scramble to pick up the pieces
painstakingly gluing my beloved pot back together

Then God drops me again
I'm shattered
and astonished that God could be so clumsy
Take care, can't you see how delicate I am
can't you see how easily I break

God picks me up with kind hands
examines me with compassion, agreeing
yes, you are exquisite, so fine, so fragile
Beautiful

God drinks from my precious pot
then breaks me again
What kind of irresponsible God is this
What careless God
breaks me open again

July 2005 (56)

UNSOLICITED ADVICE

Remember to celebrate
not just Christmas and birthdays
Take all the holidays you want
Don't miss out on anything because
you think you have to clean the house
Don't do it for the money
Scratch your creative itch
Don't wait to feel confident before you start

Spoil the ones you love
Forgive even if you can't forget
Let yourself cry at the sad bits
Graciously accept compliments
Love again, even if you're scared
Say you're sorry when you are
Smile first

Ask for what you want
Treat yourself to your favourite
Don't keep looking in the mirror
Know that you will always belong
Be kind to yourself
You don't always have to be good

Kiss a little bit longer
Don't believe everything you think
Be grateful, even on the bad days
Remember that nothing lasts forever
Lick your plate

July 2005 (57)

MY BALM

I close my eyes and sigh
and here I am
lying in the hammock of my heart
moving gently
with the softness of my breath

When I fall
from my head
past my words
I'm caught lovingly
by the hammock of my heart
and rocked to its rhythmic beat

It is my peace, my rest, my quiet
cradled in the hammock of my heart
It is constant, it is safe
to be held in the hammock of my heart

No place to go
Nothing to do
No one to please

It is my altar, my blessing, my balm
here in the hammock of my heart

July 2005 (58)

ASKING

While lying in bed this morning
I discovered the secret of how to have
what I want

I said
Sweetheart
could you please get me a big bowl
of porridge and a nice cup of tea

He smiled
and said yes
And there it was
my breakfast in bed

So I asked for a happy life
and there it was
the sun flirting with me through the window
and the morning sounds outside the door
inviting me

July 2005 (59)

LIVING A BALANCED LIFE

I know that point of balance
I swing past it all the time

August 2005 (60)

AS BEST I CAN

You are hurting
Your resentment grows
Not because I don't love you
but because I don't love you
to your precise plan

I am not a tailor-made coat
measured and sewn to fit you perfectly
I am a wild and unruly cape
fastened only to your heart

I am not just the sweet dessert
I'm the full meal
Sometimes bitter, sometimes sour
Sometimes hard to stomach

I may not always love you
to your exact requirements
I will however
keep loving you the best I can

August 2005 (61)

HIGH ON A LONELY HILL

High on a lonely hill
my self-righteous castle stands

From this lofty place
nobody can get to me
From this superior position
I am always right

Sanctimonious
upheld by my indignation
fuelled by blame
I look out over the cold grey landscape

Alone
I curl up with my smugness
forgetting that this is the cause of my loneliness
And that with this faithless friend
there is no room for love

August 2005 (62)

THINKING BETTER OF IT

Something cool and refreshing arrived today
waking me
Clear and precise
a new thought knocked on the door
So bored with those old ones
that bump around the race track inside my head

Those old frowny thoughts
chasing each other

Ah, but today
astonished
a new thought visited
popped in
and told me something that made me smile

Startled
I almost ran to lock the doors
and bolt the windows
so it wouldn't get away

Thinking better of it
I made it welcome
giving it the sunniest spot
a hot drink and lots of encouragement to stay

I even asked this new thought to invite all its friends
and together we all had a wondrous time
getting to know each other

September 2005 (63)

A TENDER WORLD AWAKES ME

This day
there is no other

The moist morning earth
awaits her lover's touch
as the sun slowly caresses the land
with his warming embrace

The breeze makes love through the trees
birds singing their consenting pleasure

A tender world awakes me
Everywhere there is only love

September 2005 (64)

GOD FELL FROM THE SKY

God fell from the sky
and unravelled before my feet

My soles touched heaven
as I stepped out across the newborn land

I walked and walked
My skin touching the moist soft grass
as the spirits played between my toes

So relieved
that at last God had fallen
from that unreachable place amongst the heavens
and had landed here in my garden
caressing my damp and human feet

God
no longer an unattainable idea
had chosen Earth

October 2005 (65)

FROM HERE I KNOW YOU

My belonging began with you
for you are my father
Yet the worlds we have inhabited
intersect only through time

I have your eyes
but I can not see you through them
I have your strong body
and still I am unable to walk in your shoes
My quick mind I gratefully inherited from you
but it does not help me to know you

My quiet heart
unspoken, familiar, recognises you
I can know you so intrinsically
and yet our differing worlds
leave rifts so great
they can only be filled by silence

Sadness, that I never really knew you
Acceptance, that I never really could
Our defining life experiences too different
no words can bridge this chasm

Your philosopher's soul
you passed down to me
From here I know you
From here
I mourn your passing

October 2005 (66)

GIRLFRIEND

When I fall, you lie down beside me
Then give me a standing ovation
when I stand up again

When I am running low
and I find my way to your door
it's snug and familiar
a soft place to land
Like melting into a favourite dressing gown
I can cuddle right in and it soothes my heart

I appreciate how you fill out the edges of my life
how you know me so well
You laugh with me as we get older
as we watch our children grow

You are my sister
my mother
my daughter

You are
my dear friend

December 2005 (67)

WORD REMEDIES

January 2006 - January 2007

A TIME WHEN

The more that people ask for copies of my writing and the more they suggest that I write a book, the more the doubt rages inside my head. It's a battle in there.

But through the turbulence, people keep on showing up to help. Like magic. A friend says "these poems are more like remedies" and I reply, "word remedies" and we both shout "Yes". A graphic designer shows up and says "I want to design and layout your writing as a book", editors show up out of nowhere. Next thing, boxes of my book, Follow Yourself Home arrive, and people start buying copies. Like magic.

THE LAST TIME

When was the last time you declared yourself innocent
without beating yourself with your guilt stick
without making yourself wrong again

When was the last time you honoured yourself
and gently said no
no apologies needed

When was the last time you clearly
asked for what you wanted
No demands, no justifications

When was the last time you lovingly
gave yourself permission

When was the last time you pleased yourself
Not others

When was the last time you were quiet with yourself
Enjoying yourself

Make this the last time you dishonour yourself

January 2006 (68)

ALWAYS THE THREAD

A fine line, a thread
weaving through our lives
Inherited strands from the ancestors
an umbilical cord from the past
Always a thread

A fragile silken filament
exquisitely embroidered on our hearts
Twisted and twirled into a thick rope
secured to the moorings

Knotted and tied into a hammock
rested and held
Sometimes a tangled net of frustration
Sometimes a string of lights in celebration

Always that thread
Intricately lacing
the earth to our bodies
our hearts to each other
to our spirit and beyond

Play with me, my friend
each of our threads
entwined and looped

Romp and leap with me
as we weave this blanket
of belonging
The very fabric of our lives

February 2006 (69)

I WAS WONDERING

All these years have passed
Do I still move you, stir you
Can I still alight your passions

If I was walking down your street
unknown
would you turn your head
curious

Sometimes
you draw me in with your eyes
and I remember our first
And I wonder
am I still your great love
am I more than the person who shares your days

If I were not here
would we have kissed enough
would your body ache towards something soft
missing me
Would we regret too many busy days
and not enough lounging love

February 2006 (70)

FILLED TO OVERFLOWING

I am not imagining this
this life filled to excess
this minute filled with this
that corner filled with that

The revealing day filled with light
Night filled with stars
strange noises and sleep

There are no spaces
no time in the day without light
no time in the night without darkness
no moment when my body doesn't feel
when my mind isn't exploring my world

No instance when I do not breathe
Every day filled with flavour
No moment when my eyes do not see
Even in silence I hear my own breathing

I am not imagining this
this feeling of fullness
spilling over into wonder

There is no time
when I am not having
the exquisite experience of living

February 2006 (71)

CLAIMED

Life is inclusive
You wake up
and here you are
included

It's you who looks out the window and gets scared
relegating yourself to the side-lines
It's you who believes you don't belong

It's those doubting voices inside your head
that have you crawling back into bed
blankets over your head
disbelieving

Life has already claimed you
each breath, proof
that existence has already
proclaimed you as its own

February 2006 (72)

THIS BLESSED BEACH

It has been a long time
since a deep distant yearning
pulled at my heart sleeve
and I remembered my way back
to this blessed beach

A long time since
a wild wind saturated my lungs
Since cold salted water
washed me
and the sun's warm hands
laid themselves on my skin

A long time
since the damp sand
made slippers on my feet
And the soothing rhythmic sound
of the sea entered me

March 2006 (73)

SWEET TIME

Time
She's nobody's sweetheart
No amount of courting
will win her over

She indulges us all
in equal measure
Wooing won't gain any extra favour

You can't save her
spend her, trick her
or waste her
Only fail to appreciate her

She's nobody's darling
sweet, sweet
precious time

March 2006 (74)

MY WANTING EARS

I found my heart
at the back of the cupboard
squashed behind
a pile of painful words

I think I need a kiss
with kindly lips
with soothing words
to flow over the wounds

Elegant droplets of kindness
falling into my wanting ears

March 2006 (75)

WHY NOT

I caught myself
daydreaming

Then said to myself
why not
So I wrote it all down
and now it's a plan

Now I know where I'm heading
and I'm taking my time

I know where I'm heading
cause I've got the plan

April 2006 (76)

I'VE COME TO LISTEN

I've come to listen
Even when it's hard

I've still come to listen

. . .

Even when I forget
and fill the listening
with my own words
I've still come to listen

Even when I'm unsure of the silence
I've still come to listen

. . .

To listen carefully
so my feet can mind the earth
And my heart can hear those hushed voices
that bring me back to here
So I can hear past my own thoughts
to distinguish you from me

Enough of my words

I've come to listen

. . .

April 2006 (77)

CELEBRATION

A celebration is gratitude expressing itself
as we joyously give our thanks

Our laughter a celebration of our delight
and our tears a celebration of our mourning

Our attention a celebration of our belonging
our actions a celebration of our believing

Our mistakes a celebration of our learning
our triumphs a celebration of our courage

Our loving a celebration of all that dwells in our heart
And at the end
our dying a celebration of our living

Have it all
Unashamedly
Celebrate it all

April 2006 (78)

TELL ME YOUR STORY

Tell me a story
Tell me your story

Tell me how you got to here
the roads that led to this moment
take me to the crossroads
show me the paths you chose

Walk me along your most treasured tracks
the tough mountains you have crossed
Show me the signposts that pointed the way
and the dead ends that left you almost defeated

And along the way
show me your summer picnic places
where happy memories still sit in the sun smiling
Share with me those secret places
where you sheltered when you were lost and adrift
Tell me of the people you loved
those who left their sweet mark
and the ones whose harshness hollowed out your heart

Recount to me all your stories
so I can know what has made you
Why some things soften your face
and others catch your breath and your eyes say no

Tell me a story
Tell me *your* story

June 2006 (79)

SELF CONSCIOUS

How do you experience me
I need to know

I need to know
so I am not forever watching myself
and wondering
am I received or am I rejected

I'm painfully aware of that anxious gap
that small space between me and the interaction
Longing to feel my acceptance
That hungry need to sink
into a deep sense of belonging

How do you experience me
I want for it to not matter
For your experience of me
to have no bearing on how I know myself

How do you experience me
I need to know
so I don't watch each moment
Looking, always looking for my wrongness
interpreting every word, every gesture

Aching to relax, simply relax
into each and every interaction

June 2006 (80)

TO CAPTIVATE MY HEART

How is it
that the exact measure of beauty
was put in your eyes
to captivate my heart
so I will never look away

How is it
that the exact music
was put into your voice
to captivate my heart
so I will never
lose you in the crowd

How is it
that the exact mixture of musk
was put upon your skin
to captivate my heart
so I will never move away

How is it
that there is an exact movement
that graces your body
to captivate my heart
so I will never let you go

July 2006 (81)

THE ANSWER TO THE QUESTIONS

Searching for the answers
That's my problem

The questions
the questions are sweet
They just sit there
relaxing
doing what questions do best
simply asking
Knowing the answers will show up
when they're ready

They always come in pairs
questions and answers
Find one and the other isn't far behind
Trick is not scaring them off
by trying too hard

Desperately searching for the answers
That's my problem

July 2006 (82)

KEEP BELIEVING

Knowing what you want
that's a problem

Believing you can have it
that's bigger problem

But to keep believing
is the biggest problem
as you want and work and wait

To keep believing
that's it
To keep believing

July 2006 (83)

MOVE SLOWLY

Move slowly towards my wounded heart

So easily does it run and hide
under the chair
behind the curtain
down the garden
lost in the trees

Coax me out
with sweet warm milk
soothing words
and a gentle touch

July 2006 (84)

BLOODY UNCOMFORTABLE

The thing about changing
is it takes you out
of your comfort zone
The thing about moving out
of your comfort zone
is that it's bloody uncomfortable

So
breathe into your belly
and stay in the discomfort
Don't try and jump out

Things will shift
Change will happen
It always does

July 2006 (85)

GOOD MORNING

I woke this morning
and found myself
accepting myself
loving myself

The boulders of self-doubt
had rolled away
and I could see for miles

August 2006 (86)

EMPTY OUT THE BLAME

Empty out the blame
That stagnant brackish water
that drowns your heart

Empty out the blame
so a fresh pure spring
can flood through you

And if the tide of resentment rises
then empty out again

November 2006 (87)

THE BLESSING OF SILENCE

The tight fist of fear
squeezes the juice from my heart
as I terrorise myself with my own thoughts
leaving no place for solace or loving

Until I lay myself down in the soft grass
and watch the trees dance unhurried in the breeze

As the clouds meander across the sky
I surrender
awakening to the blessing of a silent mind

January 2007 (88)

LIVE TODAY

Don't live this day
as if it were your last

Live today as if it were the blueprint
for your children's lives
Knowing you only have
this one day to pass on to them

Fill it with everything
you know to be true
Every treasure that you would want
your children to have and to inherit

January 2007 (89)

KEEPING ME COMPANY

This happiness
came from nowhere
Not from this or that or from you

This happiness
just hung around
and kept me company

When my day tried
to busy and bustle me along
This happiness suggested
that I hold on tightly
to her hand

January 2007 (90)

CHANGING

February 2007 - July 2009

A TIME WHEN

The magic stops and my life as I know it, vanishes. My relationship breaks down, which means my business is over and my business is also my home. My friends and family take care of me until I am ready to start a new life. I walk the hills reflecting on the life I have just lost, which helps me imagine what might come next.

AMBUSHED

The mid-life-type crisis arrives
Unannounced
Inconvenient

An ambush

All those whispered
'I'll do it one day's start to shout
The routines begin to weep
and the foundations shudder

Gripping tight, still holding on
we smile through our exhaustion
still hoping it will not happen

But the cracks keep exposing
and the shaking still threatens

The old stories can no longer
patch our life together
It's time to go down
to what is left undone
Begin to dismantle
all that we thought was so important

We don't yet know how
but we most definitely know
what we must do

August 2007 (91)

JUST FOR LISTENING

I would like three heads please
One to think with
one to speak with
and another
just for listening

It's tiring trying
to think and talk and listen
with just one head

August 2007 (92)

IT IS FOR ME

From its winter freeze
the icy heart melt begins
and love starts to flow

Fresh new water
pours from the lonely mountains
down through the quiet valleys
moving over warming rocks and rich earth

Winding through the plains
warmed in the sun
curling its way here
to awaken my body
and bathe my aching heart

And to my surprise
this spring flood
of utterly tender love
is not for another
It is for me

August 2007 (93)

ANOTHER BEAUTIFUL DAY

Another beautiful day
given into my hands
to make with what I want

Another beautiful day
offering itself
in this perfect place

Another beautiful day
has arrived
announcing
that this gift
is just for me

August 2007 (94)

NOT TO WORRY

You don't need to worry
It hasn't happened yet

And if it does
you'll be too busy
dealing with it
to worry

August 2007 (95)

TRUSTING OUR WAY

On our way to closer friendship
sometimes we'll bang into each other
drop a word into an old wound
poke a finger into a tender spot

Reminder of what is still left
sore and awkward within us

The only thing we can do
is trust our way through the hurt
Step forward and soften
moving gracefully
through the conflict

Breathing and believing
the best in each other

October 2007 (96)

TOUCHSTONE

We all need a touchstone
A place that touches us deeply
that leads us back
to ourselves

Where just the memory of the land
calls to us from afar

A place that our body recognises
and our heart remembers

December 2007 (97)

THE FINAL INJUSTICE

I am not afraid of dying
Not yet anyway

I am however
troubled by thoughts
of missing out
All those many things
that will dare to happen
without me

The final injustice
Life going on
without me

December 2007 (98)

THE TRUTH ABOUT MYSELF

I am already
all these good things
lovely, loveable, loving

Anything else I tell myself
is a lie

Every day I cleanse myself
not of any sin
but of the contaminating thought
that I am broken

I am waking from the delusion
that I am not good enough
that I am not enough

Talking back to those damaging voices
left raging inside my head

Looking into the mirror of my innocence
and seeing the sweet smile of relief
play on my face
and rest into my eyes

December 2007 (99)

A BITTER STAIN

Betrayal lives on the other side of truth
The thing not said
will forever be too late

Betrayal is not always in the deed
Betrayal is also in the secret
the cowardice of omission

With every denial
with each confessional moment lost
the wound of betrayal deepens
long before the truth is even known

Each lies
each truth withheld
leaves a bitter heart-stain
the shadow of which
takes a long time
to fade into forgiveness

December 2007 (100)

LULLABY FOR A GROWN UP

I have softened the lights
closed the doors
and pulled all the plugs

Rest your head right here
I have something to tell you

It's time to stop
You no longer need to believe
those damning and demanding voices
- your own or others'

Time to untangle the net
of every expanding choice

There is nothing for you
to do, to fix, to say, to decide

It's quiet
It's still
It is yours

December 2007 (101)

I WANT MY HEART BACK

I want my heart back

Having given it away
in some pointless bargain
I have abandoned myself

Distraught
I have tried to fill this empty heart space
with any poor substitute

I want my heart
warm and full inside

Then it can overflow
to share with another

December 2007 (102)

IT DOESN'T MATTER

It doesn't matter
if I do or if I don't
if I stop or keep going
if I stay or if I go

There is no such thing
as a destined destination
a single purposeful purpose

All there is
is experience
This choice leads to these experiences
that choice leads to those experiences

It really doesn't matter

January 2008 (103)

SURRENDERED

My tea cools beside me
as I sit down to stress

I watch the wind dance through the long grass
which needs mowing since last I looked
The washing drying in the breeze
as the sun strolls from cloud to cloud

All around me
life is happening without effort
And here I am
in the middle
incessantly trying
struggling with this
urgency about that

Overlooking the uncomplicated fact
that life is already happening

Foolishness still prevails
as I try not to try

January 2008 (104)

THE COURAGE TO SPEAK

Yes, I was hurt
A child, abused and alone

If I do not speak of it
If shame holds my tongue
then I remain complicit
and this quiet curse continues

Consent by silence
allows these wretched things
to happen
to still happen
to the young and tender

The first thing to be done
is to speak of it

So yes, I was hurt
A child, abused and alone

April 2008 (105)

LEFT BEREFT

I should have known by his lazy touch
but I married him anyway

Forgetting to expect
I hoped instead

And when love didn't come
I was left bereft
But not surprised

May 2008 (106)

FOR MYSELF

I am not defined
by how others see me

The earth does not say
"the sun does not love me"
when its warmth is muted by the cloud

When autumn leaves cover the ground
the grass does not say
"I am no longer important"

The mamaku standing tall in the forest
does not wilt from lack of praise
It knows that it is grand
doesn't need to be told

I too
am defined
By myself
For myself

May 2008 (107)

EVEN MY MIND ESCAPES

In the soft stillness of silent solitude
my heart overflows
into this soothing expanse

Billowing breaths touching everything
the greenness of a delicate fern
the quietness of the shadowing dawn
the endlessness of flowing water

And for these few moments
even my mind escapes

May 2008 (108)

THIS PLACE CALLED SUCCESS

I see you striving
and wonder
where it all leads

So much devoted effort
I see you striving
and wonder
if this place called success
even exists

I see your wide-eyed expectation
of a life full to the brim
with achieving, with accomplishment
prosperity and promise

And I wonder
what will happen
when all the striving
leads to strife
And all the wanting
leaves you wanting

June 2008 (109)

SMILING BACK

Being strong is not being a rock
hard and unbreakable

It's all the pieces left behind
when everything falls apart

It's loving the mirror and smiling back
accepting all the reflections
even when we don't know who we are anymore
even when we don't know what to do

Strength is a living membrane
responding to the moment
No longer arguing with what is

Bearing to stay in that place
of not knowing

December 2008 (110)

MAKING BAD DEALS

Making bad deals
as I trade myself for approval

Letting my need for love
override my self-respect
Trading my integrity for love

I'm putting a sign on my heart
'Not for Sale or Lease'
to remind myself
that my heart is to be shared

Never to be traded

December 2008 (111)

THE PROMISE

When I committed to you
I promised to give it everything

I believed in that promise with all my heart

Now
as things fall apart
I must blame you
Otherwise my best wasn't good enough
Otherwise I can't trust my own heart

And if I allow that to be remotely true
where might that lead

Where might that lead

December 2008 (112)

WITH JUST ONE BREATH

I forgot to breathe
Not the dying kind of not-breathing

But the kind of not-breathing
that comes from distraction
Absent
ignoring where I am
neglecting what I'm doing

The kind of not-breathing
that happens when I'm too busy out-there
and lose touch with in-here

The kind of not-breathing
that opens the door
for anxiety and mistrust

Until the moment I notice
And with that awakening nudge
I'm back
Stirred from my unconsciousness
aware of myself in this place, now

With just that one breath
I am delivered back to here

July 2009 (113)

BLOSSOMING

August 2009 - April 2014

A TIME WHEN

A friend suggests that I see this as a time to write full time, live in a caravan and eat cabbage and rice. But I don't have the courage to trust in life as a struggling writer and instead put all my effort into creating a new business. My writing falls into the well of forgetting. I'm happy. This new life is pretty damn good.

SWEET SILENCE

When the complaints
have talked themselves
into a tiresome stupor

When the old stories are bored
even with themselves
And blame can find no one to listen

When the drama has finally
played itself out

All that is left is stillness

The sweetest silence

March 2010 (114)

I SLEPT WITH MYSELF LAST NIGHT

I slept with myself last night
arms and legs outstretched
touching the sides of my own silence

Without fiction or fancy
I was only a little afraid
of the solitary darkness

Tonight I may again arch slightly
longing towards some ghostly
or imagined someone

Or I may sleep well with myself
curled up in the wonder and comfort
of my own heartbeat

Lying in my own bed
with my own body
my own thoughts

In this
my own life

March 2010 (115)

I'D RATHER

I'd rather
look at the landscape at the beach
than a pretty picture on a wall
Walk in the park than through an art gallery
Enjoy it than Facebook it
Do it than watch it

I'd rather
play music badly
than listen to it expertly played
Eat what I've grown
than something fancy I can't pronounce
Make it than buy it

I'd rather
leave my phone behind and risk missing out
than take it with me, hoping
Miss a call than miss what's happening
Be with you than txt you

I'd rather
be by myself than try too hard to be with others
Get hurt than close my heart
Walk in the dark than be scared of it
Risk being embarrassed
than be compelled to prove I'm right

April 2013 (116)

A NEW LIFE

April 2014 - December 2015

A TIME WHEN

My life is stable again. I have a new home, my business is going well, and most importantly, I meet my now-husband. My focus is split between falling for him and working in the business.

I realise I want to understand climate change more and decide to read a couple of books. Twenty eight books later, and I've finally got my head and heart around it. Not only does this lead me back to my writing table, it also pushes me out into the world to advocate for climate change action. Words come back and my creativity is here to stay. I'm happy and grateful.

THIS GIVEN TIME

I don't arrive in places like this very often
This given time

Time alone
not rushing through

Delight in the honesty of my own style
nothing side-lined
Me in the middle
in the corners, in the garden, on the couch
through the door, in the mirror

My loving arms around my life
sweet words whispered to my own goodnights

I don't arrive in places like this very often
This given time
Time alone

April 2014 (117)

BREADCRUMB TRAILS

Already

Already I have let myself
go beyond any place
I have ever allowed my heart
to venture before

I have wandered so far
into love's enchanted forest
that I have forgotten to be scared
of the witches, the bad wolves
and all the other traps
set for an innocent heart

The old love stories tell me
there may be no way back
The navigation star
is lost on a clouded night
The breadcrumb trails
have all been eaten

I'd heard about these hidden doors
that lead us into forgotten gardens
Until we get so lost
that we never want to be found again

June 2014 (118)

PLAYING HIDE AND SEEK WITH THE PAST

Today
those old memories
found me again
Tracking me down
and reminding me of
the long-buried past

I indulged in a few
of my favourite distractions
all the while knowing
they could not save me

I got lost
playing hide and seek
with the past

And finally
I had to admit
that I am still afraid
of those old cold ghosts

They can still reach through
from the past
and catch me

August 2014 (119)

OUR DARLING PLANET

It's a new disease, the experts say

From a distance she looks well enough
But up close, up close

She has a low-grade temperature
and all the indications are
that it will turn into a raging fever

Her waters are becoming acidic
and she's retaining fluid

She has open sores and hard crusty scabs
She's not as beautiful as she once was

And some times she can hardly breathe

She's ailing
She's tired
Our darling planet

September 2014 (120)

NO MORE ALIBIS

It's not fair

I'm not talking about myself
I've fully-lived a comfortable life
Couldn't have asked for more

It's not fair
that I've taken more than my share
and left behind more than I should
But it is done
My carbon load is out there
joining in the warming
of the global commons

I did not know
that my choices
would leave a legacy
that cannot be undone

But truthfully
I had an inkling
That it was all too convenient
disposable, dislocated
All too good to be true

And now I do know
Bare, stark
No more excuses
No more alibis

September 2014 (121)

ON A COLLISION COURSE WITH REALITY

We can't negotiate with climate change
We don't get to decide who will win and who will lose

This is a non-negotiable
unwinnable argument
with the callous laws of physics and chemistry

There are no swings and roundabouts
no happily balanced seesaw
only a slide leading to a place
where none of us want to go

This is not about
who's wrong
our country or your country
or our history
or your rights or our needs
or which ideology
or my version
or who has it the hardest

It's about the humbling reality
of what is actually happening

And what it will take

October 2014 (122)

ON EVERY ACCOUNT

The planet's going bankrupt
with banks still full of pretend wealth

It's business as usual
as the earth slowly goes out of business

We are overdrawn on every account
with no means of clearing our debt

No duty of care from our leaders
no stewardship
Business only minding its own self-serving business
Experts shelling out advice
selling us out to the highest bidder

And no excuse from the rest of us
for blindly accepting what is not ours

For receiving stolen goods

December 2014 (123)

NOT ALL CARBON IS EQUAL

The carbon produced
to feed a family
is worth more
than the carbon that comes out
the back of a jet ski

The fuel to drive to work
has more validity
than the fuel needed
for a trip to Bali

The energy used
to simply live a decent life
is more justified
than all this excess

December 2014 (124)

STUFFED

All this stuff
All this effort
All this busyness

It hasn't worked
We are no happier
than we were decades ago

We are so damn busy
Managing time as if it were manageable
Stuffed to overflowing with stuff
Progressing progress

And all we have more of
is effort
activity
and endless incessant stuff

December 2014 (125)

VAGUELY AWARE

I open my front door
and take a moment
Everything seems to be fine

Closing the door
I drift through my day
vaguely aware that something
is not quite right

Vaguely aware that the roses
are budding in winter
Vaguely aware that I used to stomp
on frozen puddles when I was a child

Vaguely aware that I
should be doing something
Something about this feeling
that something's not quite right

February 2015 (126)

TOO BIG TO FAIL

We bailed out big banks
We bailed out big business
We even bailed out a country or two

How about the planet?

Who is going to bail out the planet?
Pluto?
Mars?
God?
The garden pixies?

March 2015 (127)

MAGICAL THINKING

I would even believe in God
if I thought it would help

Any kind of magical thinking will do

March 2015 (128)

AN INSURMOUNTABLE MOUNTAIN

An insurmountable mountain
of resistance
of distraction
of denial

Outright denial
It's not happening

Impact denial
It won't be that bad

Responsibility denial
Someone else will sort it

Protective denial
Hiding from despair, overwhelm, fear

Wishful thinking denial
Something good is bound to happen

Suspicious denial
You go first

Magical thinking denial
God, the universe, mother nature will save us

Liability denial
It's their fault, not mine

Tech denial
Super hero technology to the rescue

Distraction denial
I recycle, I use green products

Busyness denial
Too tired, too busy, too much

So
We are stuck
up against this
insurmountable mountain of denial

Looking for the tiniest crack
the smallest crevice

A place where we can finally begin

April 2015 (129)

SIMPLE ARITHMETIC

Something has got to give
or somethings going to break

As we keep going
on our merry-go-round
of endless growth

We measure it, predict it
expect it, accept it
A system dependent on
on continuous consumption
on a definitively finite planet

The simplest arithmetic
tells me that this
simply doesn't add up

June 2015 (130)

MY BIG CARBON BOOTS

What needs to happen
for me to admit
That this includes me

What is the tipping point
that will trip me up
knock me over
wake me up

When will I stop stomping around
in my big carbon boots

When do I say to myself
Enough

August 2015 (131)

CLIMATE CHANGE

Go Away

I don't want to talk
I don't want to think
I don't want to know

It's too hard

August 2015 (132)

FAR TOO FAR

Far too clever
to be smart enough
to know we've got it wrong

We've gone far too far
to accept
that we need a reboot

Far too many
reasonable reasons
excusable excuses
justifying justifications

Far too far
from what is so
excruciatingly important

Our expectant children
Our innocent planet
Our tender humanity

October 2015 (133)

IT'S NOT

Thinner than the skin of an apple
thinner even than the dust on the shelf

Between the enormity
of endless space
and the crust of the earth
is a tiny, thin
breathtakingly sheer layer

Our atmosphere is where
all that we love and cherish exists

And even more delicate
is the flimsy canvas of soil and rock and sea
The place where we love and sleep, eat and play
and believe that all things are possible

Acting as if
these bountiful oceans are boundless
They aren't

Acting as if
the very soil that feeds us
stays magically stable and fertile
It doesn't

Acting as if
this layer of precious air
is impervious, indestructible
that it is infinitely supportive of us

It's not

October 2015 (134)

ANYTHING EXCEPT

Just ask us about our children
Our grandchildren
Real or imagined

Ask us what we would do
to protect them
Ask us what we would do
to give them the best life

The answer is
anything
Everything

Then ask us about climate change
We'll duck, deflect, distract
We'll squirm

We will do anything for our children
Anything except
engage with climate change
personally or collectively

November 2015 (135)

WHEN WE WENT TO PARIS

It's like deciding to lose weight
while refusing to get off the couch
Like making a cake
without turning on the oven
Doing the washing
without hanging it on the line

Good intentions
but meaningless

Like world leaders deciding on
two degrees maximum global temperature increase
but having no actual plan
no accountability
with most of the effort going into back-pedaling

We have confused
intention for result
activity for achievement
a resolution for a solution
a meeting for an accord
a press statement for a binding agreement

We have confused
talking about it
with doing it

December 2015 (136)

I WANT MY OLD CLIMATE BACK

I want things the way they were
I want my old climate back

I don't want there to be a lag time
years of warming already in the pipeline
this unrelenting legacy

I don't want the climate
to change any more

I want my old climate back

December 2015 (137)

HOW DO I BEAR IT

The knowing
the disbelief
the aching grief

Screaming into the collective silence
numb, passive, mute

Overwhelmed by the enormity
humiliated by my own inaction

Up against the wall
of my own protection

December 2015 (138)

A RUNAWAY MIND

The problem with a runaway mind
is it leaves you brainless

Just when you need it to think something
your brains gone rouge
Just when you need to do something
There's nothing there

A runaway mind
tells you stories
that scare you senseless
Repeating reruns
with deadening regularity

A runaway mind
allows unwanted gatecrashers
to ruin your party
Conducting an entire chorus
of unhelpful advice

A runaway mind
is a pack of spooked horses
stampeding off in every direction

A runaway mind
is exhausting

December 2015 (139)

OUTPOURING

March and April 2016

A TIME WHEN

The words pour out. The environmental stuff breaks my heart with grief and guilt. I can hardly bear it. Writing helps. So does taking action in my own life and out in the world. I decide that it's time to put another book together.

I'M A POLITICIAN

I'm a politician
not a leader
I don't lead, I follow
I follow the money

I'm no different from you
I do what my employers asks
I get my orders from those
who give me
the money

I'm a politician
not a leader
I don't lead, I follow
I follow the money

March 2016 (140)

WHEN OUR HABITS BETRAY US

When our old habits betray us
best we find better friends
to help us on our way

Mr Will Power only works on good days
On a bad day
Mr Will Power won't get out of bed

Mrs Motivation is not always motivated
And being full of excuses
waxes and wanes and does as she pleases

However
may I introduce you to Constance Routine
an old and reliable friend

Ms Routine doesn't like sudden moves
takes things slow and steady
One small change before another

She is kind
always wanting the best for us
Constance Routine is most agreeable
always doing what she's asked

March 2016 (141)

WHEN I AM IN PAIN

In this moment
I don't need you to fix me
I don't need your sympathy or your kindly advice
Please don't try to convince me it's not so bad
or pretend that this isn't happening

To do this
leaves me
lonely, angry, invisible, ashamed

What I need most
is your acknowledgement
of my pain
of my discomfort

Ask me just one question
What do you need right now
right here

And if I can't answer
simply do something simple for me
Something nurturing
so I feel your care

March 2016 (142)

LOSING MY MIND

I don't think
I've lost it
Not really lost it

I'm sure I put it down
around here
Someplace

I'm sure it's still
waiting for me
Somewhere

March 2016 (143)

A WEE TASTE

A conversation
is a smorgasbord of ideas
having lunch together

A conversation
is where we have a wee taste
of things we don't already know

A good conversation
is a feast for the mind

March 2016 (144)

TRICKED NOT TRICKLED

The economic trickle down effect
that promised flow of wealth
It hasn't found me yet

All that talk of less tax, less regulation, free trade
has built financial dams
to hold the flow of money
for those few who re-made the rules

There never was a stream of wealth
for the rest of us

The floodgates are still holding tight
I am stranded high and dry
I've been tricked
not trickled

March 2016 (145)

THIS PERFECT DISCONNECT

We measure ourselves by our intent
knowing we mean no harm

We measure others by their impact
the harm they are causing us

This perfect disconnect
this dividing rift
means we drift even further apart

Can we bear to hear
the impact we have on others
irrespective of our intent
Holding quietly our dearly held
excuses and explanations

Can we listen to their intent
no matter how hurt
or wronged we may feel

Can we judge others
as we judge ourselves

Can we connect this disconnect
by walking across the bridge
between intention and impact

March 2016 (146)

THIN STRANDS

When the hard issues hit the political table
each party rushes off on their own
thin strand of ideology
Arguing, postulating
critical and indignant

Meanwhile
the real questions remain
Discouraged, abandoned, strangled
quietly left to fester

So much attention directed to the side shows
while the hard issues still sit
lonely in the middle of the table
knowing they will be hoisted back
used for political expediency
at the very next opportunity

March 2016 (147)

THE SUN HAS STARTED SLEEPING IN

The yellow and orange sunflowers
are almost gone from my garden
Just a few brave blooms remain

A sighed relief
that summer has had enough
of rushing about
The sun has started sleeping in
letting the birds snooze
a little longer each morning

The cooling calm at dusk
holds a promise

The winter quiet is coming
curled up warm and snug at home
The wet and cold to keep me inside
The greying dark a reminder
that it's time for rest

March 2016 (148)

THE REVOLVING DOOR

Maybe
maybe it's just
too complicated
too complex
changes too fast

What if the revolving door of restructuring
will never actually work
What if restructuring does nothing
but make us giddier and giddier
And what if this rollercoaster of change
does nothing but leave us unable to think straight

What if, not knowing what else to do
we requisition yet another restructure
on this swinging merry-go-round
of perpetual, mindless change

March 2016 (149)

A NOBLE VIRTUE

We honour ANZAC day
we remember the wartime dead
Not only because of their courage
but because we long to believe
that we would do the same
Fight selflessly for our children
willing sacrifice whatever it takes

The climate is changing
So fast - too fast for us to adapt
This strange new enemy
of our very own making

Who will we allow to call us to arms
When will the heroism begin
How far do things need to go
before we finally acknowledge
that it will take all of us pulling
with all our might

When will sacrifice once again
become the noblest of virtues

March 2016 (150)

AVOIDING HEARTACHE

I am desperately afraid of heartache

I want to control things
Watchfully anticipating
steeling myself
withdrawing
Wilfully determined

Interrupting the enjoyment of now
in a vain hope
that by being ready
I can avoid any kind of dreaded surprise

As if readiness ever stopped heartache
As if being forewarned
ever lessened the pain

March 2016 (151)

DEAR STUDENTS

Tertiary education is now a business
with vested, invested interests
who aren't that interested
in your interests

They are only interested
in your money

March 2016 (152)

NOTHING LEFT TO THINK

When I can't get my head straight
When I'm overthinking
When my thoughts disturb and interrupt

That's when I go to the beach
Inhale the tiny drops of sea caught in the wind
watch the small pebbles dance with the waves
hear the low rumble of their teasing delight
taste the bite of salt on my lips
collect tiny pieces of polished glass

And then there is nothing left to think

That's when I go to the bush
Breath the air just breathed by the birds
watch the leaves playing with the wind
inhale that deep damp fragrance after rain

And then there is nothing left to think

That's when I go to my garden
Smile back at the flowers
who are still smiling at the sun
bury my hands in the moist brown earth

And then there is nothing left to think

Sometimes I simply walk
one foot and then the other
Each step resting gently on solid ground

And then there is nothing left to think

March 2016 (153)

NOT WORKING

Sometimes things don't work out
for reasons other than
ignorance or ineptitude

Sometimes we fail
because we are attempting things
that are not possible

We drop this, it breaks
We try this, we fail
We want this, we're disappointed
We plan this, we're misguided
We think this, we're wrong

Some things
simply
aren't
possible

March 2016 (154)

NOT JUST THEM

Nobody likes to be made wrong
Not just them
us too

We can't change anyone
by making them wrong
All they will do is push back
or shut down

All we can do
is be kind and clear
Influence how they are with us
by how we are with them

March 2016 (155)

WHEN I WAS YOUNGER

When I think how wired I was
how much energy was frittered away
on emotional angst and trying too hard

When I think of the waste
All that precious liveliness
taken for granted

How careful I have become
Kinder to myself and others
and grateful

March 2016 (156)

EVEN THOUGH YOU HAVE GONE

I still know you
even though you are no longer here
You are still my beloved, my friend
even were I to commit to another

I still have a relationship with you
the things I show you
our conversations inside my head
the continuing stories from our shared past

What was once companionship between two
has become my sacred internal communion

March 2016 (157)

MANNERS MONITOR

I'm off to parliament
to teach our politicians
some manners

No running the country
until they can be polite

A star for good behaviour
Five stars and they get a certificate
to take back to their electorate

No talking over, calling names
put downs, accusations
pretend questions or smart-arse comments

Once they've learnt how to play nicely
then they can run the country

March 2016 (158)

LOVE TAKES ITS TIME

True love can only ever come slowly
No matter how much we want
to hurry through to safe ground

It takes time to find
the securing glue of shared memories
of enough living together
to join two lives

No matter how fast we want love
to knit us together
the beginning is always precarious
as we slowly twist the threads
into something that can withstand
the yanks, the wear, the loose ends
without unravelling

We can't push love any faster
than the crafty fingers of time
can weave us together

March 2016 (159)

NOT EVEN A SANDCASTLE

I want to stand on the beach
seeing this landscape as it once was

No tall, neat piles of stones
built for some spiritual effect

No moving of the long-bleached driftwood
into beach huts along the shore
Not even a sandcastle

I can ignore the dark sandy roads
and the tracks down to the beach
The holiday homes laden with summer memories
I can even block out the hungry picnic tables

I want to stand on the sand
look out and pretend that this
is nature as it was
Naked
Before we covered it
with a myriad of modifications

I want to stand on the shore
seeing only the sand, the waves
the rocks, the seaweed, the sea
the seabirds

A landscape bare of us

March 2016 (160)

IN TOO MANY WORDS

When words won't work
when they get snarled and snagged
When the meaning gets lost in all the talk
and their definition escapes

That's when we let the silence
of our simply being here
do all that is needed

Hold my hand
as we walk
Put your arms around me
as we meet
Touch my back
so I know I have done well
Stroke my head
when I am ailing
Nod your head
so I know that you know
Rub my cheek
as I wake
Caress me
so I feel your care
Point the way
when I am lost
Hold me tight
when grief takes hold
Smile generously
when I walk through the door
Stand up for me
when I can't do it for myself
but sit down again
when I remember how

Touch me
Quietly
March 2016 (161)

IN PRAISE OF BLOKES

One day all the blokes and blokettes will be gone
and nothing will ever be fixed again

Unappreciated
in this age
of easy acquisition
easy disposal
revolving fashions of superficial innovation
Obsolescence around every bend

The younger ones
have little need
to learn the skills, the crafts
to master the tools of the repairing trade
Too busy with the next new thing

One day all the fixers will be gone
and nothing will ever be fixed again

March 2016 (162)

THE SCIENTISTS HAVE GOT IT WRONG

I want them to be wrong
I want for this not to be true

I want to still believe
that resources are unlimited
that our lives of comfort and privilege
are unending
with no strings
no small print

And what do I find
The scientists have got it wrong
that it is far worse
moving far quicker
than the scientists had predicted

And against this
unrelenting mountain is evidence is
flawed analysis
willful blindness
wishful thinking

March 2016 (163)

I HAD ALWAYS KNOWN

Deep down
I had always known
my Love would come

But in my impatience
I agreed too soon
and said yes to someone else's loving
Or maybe I was just too scared to wait

Then again
if we had met back then
would we have recognised each other
could our younger selves have known

Now
you are here
My Love has come

March 2016 (164)

WHAT COUNTS

How much you earn has little bearing on
how important your work is
how much you contribute
even how hard you work

It tells nothing about your heart
or the emotional wake you leave behind
Whether people grow and expand in your presence
or feel deflated and diminished

How much you earn
does not reflect
how responsible you are
for the full effects of your actions
What motivates you beyond
your reputation and how much you own

What you earn
measures everything
except what counts

March 2016 (165)

AT ANY COST

Holding on to my privilege
with one hand
while grabbing for more
with the other

I believe I deserve more
Believe it is my right
and believe in this right at all costs

At the cost of those more vulnerable
The cost of the young and those not yet born
At the cost of the delicate systems of life

At any cost
Any but my own

March 2016 (166)

GETTING CLOSE ENOUGH

How do I let the knowledge
of climate change
close enough so that I understand it
that I get it

How do I let it touch me
in such a way
that I feel the risk

How do I bear to feel
my own culpability
so I change

How do I let it get to me
so that I am compelled to do something

Without falling
into despair and unable to act
Without falling
into delusion and no need to act
Without falling
into inadequacy and losing faith in myself
Without falling
into distraction and doing the wrong things
Without falling
into fantasy and believing false prophets
Without falling
into blame and pointing the finger
Without falling
into shame and hide away
Without falling
into wishful thinking and believing in miracles

How do I get close enough to understand
without becoming overwhelmed
into inaction

March 2016 (167)

FROM MY VIEW OF THE WORLD

If I lived in a world of one
everything would make sense
to me

But I live in a world
with all of you
Believing in the rightness of
of my own view
and the likely delusion of yours

Crammed in closer and closer
connected yet disconnected
constantly merging, colliding
acting, interacting, reacting

Fortified behind my own view
refusing to acknowledge yours

March 2016 (168)

FOR DEAR LIFE

Don't teach our children that
they can do anything, everything
Stop teaching them about success

Teach them instead how to take
care of themselves
amid this uncertain
change and turmoil

Teach them how to grieve
for the world that should
have been theirs
Before the climate changed
before life became even more
complicated

Teach them to be grateful
for each good thing
And to know how to distill
what still remains true
and to stay faithful

And most of all
teach them about failure
The acceptance of a battle lost
and the ability to keep going
in the face of sure defeat

Teach them how to hold on
to what is dear
And to hold on
for dear life

March 2016 (169)

SNEAKING UP ON MYSELF

Everything I need
is right here

All I need do
is look a little closer
Creep around the corner
quietly
sneakily
and catch it quick

Before my wanting heart
my critical brain
my restless mind
takes over

March 2016 (170)

EATING OURSELVES ALIVE

I want, I want, I want, I want
That's what marketing does

Makes us into wanting machines

Consuming stuff
Gobbling debt
Devouring precious resources

A snake feeding on its own tail
we are eating ourselves alive

March 2016 (171)

DON'T LET THEM WIN

Do whatever it takes to mend yourself
The childhood abuse, the neglect
it was not your fault

Don't let blame or shame
stop you from putting
yourself back together
From clearing away the debris
left behind

If you don't
If what happened then
tarnishes what happens now
Then they will have won
They will have won

March 2016 (172)

THE EMOTIONAL FILING CABINET

Get off your high horse
Sell off the high moral ground
Decommission the complaints department
Stop trying to balance the books

Empty out the emotional filing cabinet

They didn't get out of bed this morning
simply to get up your nose
Their story about you
sounds just as compelling
as your story about them

Empty out the emotional filing cabinet

March 2016 (173)

DEAR MARKETING

Stop feeling up my feelings
unfastening my security straps
Trying to get to my most vulnerable places
exploiting any weakness

You are nothing but a dandy
not to be trusted
With your noisy buzz
your flashy clothes
and your sweet-talking sly words
Constantly trying to wheedle
your way into my wallet
With all your tricks
to make me buy your stuff

Colonizing every spare space in my head
and every other space besides
You'll do anything to coax me
into your seductive game

Stop stalking me
Get out of my face
Stop interrupting me
Be quiet

I can decide for myself
who I am, what I need
and when I want it

Yours sincerely
The reluctant consumer

March 2016 (174)

CONSUMPTION

Consumption used to be
a disease people died from
We cured it

Then we created
a new and more deadly form

A systemic disease
creeping over
our lands, our seas
through the air
through our bodies
and into our minds

This new disease tricks us
into attacking ourselves
Feeding an insatiable need
greed for more of everything

The cure
no magic pill

The cure
to practice moderation and simplicity
to remember to be grateful
to know how to make-do

March 2016 (175)

CONFLICT OF SELF INTEREST

How can I possibly see over
my own privilege
from this safe, warm, full-bellied
advantage point

How can I look back at myself
How can I continue to be
a feel-good liberal

Ignoring
my complicit participation
in a system
that keeps me
safe, warm and full-bellied

March 2016 (176)

SO BUSY BEING BUSY

It happened again

I fell into the great well of forgetting
lost in lists, demands and worry
Too busy being busy

I got caught up in the doing
and forgot what I was doing it for

Climbing up the ladder
only works if it is against the right wall
Ticking off the list
if it achieves something I still believe in
Finishing the plan
if I end up somewhere that matters

So very busy being busy

March 2016 (177)

SEEING PAST ME

There is nothing out there
Only me in here
looking out through masked eyes
perceiving, judging, interpreting

There is nothing out there
that is not seen by me in here

Imprinted on my eyes
are all the many things
I have seen before
Leaving their obscuring points and patterns

Only through curious and careful eyes
can I see past me
to the faintest, tiniest glimpse
of what might actually be out there

March 2016 (178)

LEFT WANTING

I see you striving
and I wonder
where it all leads
So much devoted effort

I see you striving
and wonder
if this place called success
even exists

I see your wide-eyed expectation
of a life full to the brim
with achieving, with accomplishment
prosperity and promise

And I wonder
what will happen
When all the striving
leads to strife
And all the wanting
leaves you wanting

March 2016 (179)

WHEN YOUR STUFFING FALLS OUT

When childhood knocks
the stuffing out of you

You look out
at the great picture of life
and you can't see yourself

When you go off looking
for your place of belonging
and can't find yourself anywhere

Until the day
you find yourself
just where you were abandoned

And holding your own hand
you venture out to claim for yourself
had which had been stolen

April 2016 (180)

WHAT SHALL I BE

I asked my dad once
"What do you think I should do when I leave school"
"Whatever you want, dear"
I didn't know how to know what I wanted

I told me Mother
"I think I'd like to got to broadcasting school"
"What makes you think you could do that"
I was so untested in my seventeen year old world
that I didn't know how to answer

I told my friend
"I think I'll be a teacher"
"You'd be lousy at that"
I didn't know enough to ask her how she knew

So I asked the guidance counsellor
for some guidance
"I think you should be a teacher"
I hit a confused dead end

I went to university and tried on a few things
Until I asked myself why
With no decent answer, I quit

So I put a pack on my back and hitch-hiked
my way through life, doing whatever found me
Mostly I enjoyed myself
Mostly it was good and I paid my way

Meanwhile, I asked an interested man
"What should I do with my life"
"Marry, me and come and live mine"
So I carefully, cunningly avoided the question
by living somebody else's life

But the question still sat there
"what to do when I grow up"
Then at last the answer found me
That thing you have always longed for
"that you believed you could never have"

April 2016 (181)

WAIT MY DARLING CHILDREN

When you marry Safety and Security
the safe haven inevitably becomes a trap
Or the endless boredom
means you eventually make
a tedious escape

When you marry Passion
You're dizzy and giddy
swinging from ecstasy to despair
Overcome with exhaustion
as you crawl away in embarrassed defeat

When you marry Money and Status
You shamefully dislike yourself
but snobbishly despise them more
Finally you rebel or are expelled
taking away as much collateral as you can carry

When you marry Duty
you are crushed under the obligation
as you disappear into dulled conformity
Or live out your life-sentence
spiting, spitting, swiping
resenting

When you marry Habit
laziness means you forget to choose
Your life waltzes past
in a monotonous but adequate blur
and you never quite get around to leaving

So wait my darling children
Wait until being with them brings out
what you most like about yourself
When resolving conflict
is a mutual discovery
When they make you laugh
and you don't have to try so hard

April 2016 (182)

THIS COURTSHIP WITH ENOUGH

I want to keep
my life right here
Grateful for all I have
wishing for nothing more

I don't want a life
any bigger than I have
I am content with this life
deep with naïve simplicity

I am loving
this calm
this quiet
Looking with soft eyes
and taking my time

This permission
I have given myself

This courtship with enough

April 2016 (183)

BEING EQUALLY KIND

It's not easy to answer
when our instant, exhausting response
is invariably yes

Unwilling to disappoint
we never quite know who to help first

How to be kind to the other
and equally kind to ourselves

April 2016 (184)

WHOSE MEDIA?

Our media?

A curious cat
or a fat cat?

A watch dog
or a lap dog?

In our interest
or their own monied self-interest?

April 2016 (185)

YOU HOWEVER

Not you
You've always been brave enough
to be your same self
no matter who is in the room

Not me
I often feel unacceptable
so offer up subtly modified versions of myself
in the hope of keeping safe

You however
delight in the solitary me
the me that hangs around
when I am on my own

April 2016 (186)

MY ORPHANED IMAGINATION

In truth
when I began
it was impossible
My longing was a dark fugitive
My imagination orphaned
in this grown-up world

With sincerity and resolve
I began to write
one right word and then another
One small act of self-rebellion at a time

From the dark shadows of my imagination
my words escaped
and found their way here
To this page

My words found their way home
to me
The writer

April 2016 (187)

I WILL NOT ASK

I want you to want to
I don't want to ask

If you really loved me
you would know
If you really loved me
I wouldn't have to ask

I want you to be the adult
and know what I want
And I want to be the child
and not have to ask

I may sulk
I may snipe

But I will not ask

April 2016 (188)

I SIMPLY FORGET

Before you
my real life was always being alone

Even with the ones I truly love
I'm still being mother, companion, advisor
Even if just a little

After the busyness, after the activity
after the conversation, after the experience
I would find myself again
in my solitude
With nobody, nothing
to second guess

But with you
I simply forget
Even when you are in the room
even when you are lying next to me
even when we are holding hands
even in the kiss
even when I doubt

With you
I simply forget

April 2016 (189)

HELPING MYSELF FEEL BETTER

I'll have a trim latte
and a piece of cinnamon cake please

Would you like cream
or yoghurt with that

Both please

April 2016 (190)

COLLECTING TIME

Once upon a time
we collected signatures of
famous and admired people
A perfect secret for our
treasured top drawer

Now we take selfies with anyone
remotely famous and not necessarily admired
And with one click
we announce it to the world
or anyone who might possibly notice

April 2016 (191)

DISTANCE BLINDNESS

I wander about the leafy, tree-lined streets
with their happily polished door handles
tenderly tended gardens

It's hard to remember
that there are things we never see
That much is so desperately wrong

That there are other harsh and less happy places
where people and the planet
are stripped bare of dignity
are ill-fated and luckless
are gutted for the pleasure and comfort
of the few

That's us
We who live in safe and prettied houses
Skim-reading and actively ignoring the reports
of such destruction, of such despair

With the luxury of believing
it could never happen to us
or to ours
Forgetting
that this planet belongs to us all

That the blindness of distance and distraction
does not make us
innocent
or safe

April 2016 (192)

BIG IMPORTANT PEOPLE

Little mice really do scurry
I just spied one hurrying
across the path
where I walk in the trees

Big important people stomp
especially when you get too close
and clomp when they don't get their way

Just spied a whole herd of them
stampeding through the streets
That was on my other walk through the town

April 2016 (193)

ALMOST FORGOTTEN

Tucked away in a corner
behind the have-tos and the everyday
are some ideals and ideas we once held so close

Now and then
we need to go down
and have a good rummage
to remember what's important
Don't wait for the crisis

It's already getting late

All those things put away for later
in those safe
almost forgotten places
Time to make sure nothing
is left out or left behind

Time for a good sort out
Time to make space

April 2016 (194)

FRUSTRATING

May 2016 - March 2018

A TIME WHEN

I come to the realisation that the ease with which Follow Yourself Home came together was a fluke. I'm struggling with this new book. I can't find the right structure, I rewrite and rewrite and it's still not working. I start the hunt for an editor. Frustration leads to distraction and I come to accept that this yo-yoing between the writing flowing and getting stuck is part of the creative life.

OFF YOU GO

I want you to be kind
to yourself

No, not when
you're ready

Earlier than that
Off you go

June 2016 (195)

MY HURTING HEART WON'T LISTEN

I get a fright
I get scared
I become anxious and uncertain

Understanding is usually enough
but sometimes my head
can't convince my heart
to listen
or to trust

I fret
trying to remind myself
of all the love and goodness

But still my hurting heart
won't listen

June 2016 (196)

TO THE PROMISED LAND

After everything
we still got ourselves caught in this trap
of big business, big money
big growth, big bullshit

Pirated and polished politics
Bought and biased media
Forced and fictional pop culture
Frantic and rampant consumerism
Corrupt and bloated food

Nature commoditised
carved up into saleable potions
hocked off to the next besotted bidder

Dazed and dulled down
We are stuck in this mindless rush
to the promised land

July 2016 (197)

PUSHING AGAINST EACH OTHER

When our views don't like each other
and we both want our own way
When I push
please push back

Not so hard
that I fall over, flattened
Just hard enough
that I know where you stand

Don't give in either
leaving me in mid-air
I need to know
you are firmly there

As we push against each other
as we rock between our positions
we form a swaying yet stable base

Knowing where each the stands
we can trust in our differences

July 2016 (198)

RESPONSIBILITY

If your liability is limited
where does the rest of it go

August 2016 (199)

STORIES

There are two sides to every story
Not just ours

August 2016 (200)

SUCH DANGEROUS THINGS

There is a wee hole
in the lattice of my wellbeing
That intricate lacy scaffolding
that keeps me upright and whole

And through such a tiny gap
can crawl
belly first
such dangerous things

Those daunting doubting winds
that whistle through
in the dark of night
leaving distrust and haunting suspicion

Those silent stinging comments
that leave raw, red welts of misgiving

And through these smallest of cracks
those wheedling roots of weedy thoughts
plant themselves in my heart
and grow furiously in the rain

September 2016 (201)

SUCH A TREAT

A body alive
with sensation
Hands to hold
legs to dance
hunger to feed
eyes to explore
skin to feel

A heart to do
all the wondrous things
that only hearts can do

A mind so peculiar, so private as to
contemplate anything and everything

All of this
for the whole of my life

A world indulgent with play

September 2016 (202)

WAKE ME LIKE THIS

When I irritate you
when I do those things
that hurt
that undermine

Remember that I am asleep
dead to the world of those around me
stumbling and lost
somewhere old and troubled

Be kind and rouse me gently
as I am charging about
in an old and murky dream
and I have forgotten to be kind to you

Wake me like this
as you ease me back through
these hard and unforgiving walls
Bring me back to my real and loving life

And forgive me
as I may fall asleep again

September 2016 (203)

THIS SMALL WORLD IS ENOUGH

A dusk walk along the still wild shore
after days of storm
And these shaky isles
have been rocking and quaking too

On one side of the road, the houses are finishing their day
on the other
the waves are tumbling head-first into the shore
The day is over but the night has not yet taken charge
The colours have faded
but the shapes and their moving are still sharp and keen

The lone evening star has arrived between
the folds of corrugated cloud
Nobody – nothing – owns this time
It is the witching hour when the
incurably curious cats appear from nowhere

It's at times like this that I almost believe
in ghosts and goblins, fairies and angels
Worldly things cannot find me
I no longer care about decisions, about Donald
about earthquakes or the floods

The eerie air I breathe is more alive
A duet of day and night sounds reach my ears
and my body feels strangely more my own
I find a fullness in my unfolding heart
even the other twilight walkers feel like kin

I savour the majesty more than the madness
happy with my place in the shambles of living

This small world is enough for me
At least until morning

September 2016 (204)

WONDERING AT THE WONDERS

I am deeply fascinated by the holes
dug through the pavements and the streets

A reminder that below us is always earth
microbes and history and old roots
There were trees and grasses
creatures and streams and such

Don't get me wrong
I am most grateful
for roads and tap water and plugs and phones
All the privileges that raw-nature does not need

Sometimes
when I look into these open holes
I wonder at the wonders
we have buried and lost

October 2016 (205)

WHEN I STOP INTERRUPTING MYSELF

To no longer be afraid of my own thoughts
to stop spooking myself
Scaring myself breathless
with doubt and self-judgement
To stop pushing myself around
with threats or worse

To allow soft space for silence
To be a kind and thoughtful host to the quiet
To stop interrupting myself

To spend enough kind-time with myself
so that we can become
fast friends

October 2016 (206)

I GIVE UP

I have changed my mind

You don't have to completely understand me
You don't have to know
how to give me everything I need

In the struggle to get your full agreement
everything becomes disagreeable

Therefore
I give up
I give in

October 2016 (207)

A DAILY RITUAL

Writers and artists often talk
of walks with the trees or along the shore
This daily ritual

Even if it means striding out
between downpours of winter rain
squalls of equinoctial wind
or strolling through the evening softness
after the heat of a summer day

They know all the shades
of the seasons and the weather
Intimately acquainted with each private landscape
Familiar with the drifting sounds
of waves on the rocks on each and any tide
A confidant to the birds and the people nearby
they feel deeply the changes
the comings and the goings

They know these places of belonging by heart
And from this intimate knowing
they are reminded each day
to go back home and create

October 2016 (208)

WAITING

Current wisdom asserts
that we do not dawdle
That we take things head on
be brave, be determined, forge ahead

But sometimes
hiding
running away
or taking our time
is for the best

Until we are ready
to try again
To venture out
holding on to ourselves
no matter what we may find

Permission
to have a rest, to recuperate
before starting out again
And only when we are ready

Taking all things
at our own sweet pace
to our own whispered place

November 2016 (209)

IN THE MIDDLE OF THE STREET

It wasn't just the wheels that fell off
it was everything
And I was left there
sore and naked
in the middle of a busy street

There were too many
fast moving things
and I could not find
an unlocked door
a coat big enough
a manhole
or my wings

I just stood there
excruciatingly exposed

Nobody came
Maybe it was my own fault
but still
nobody came

November 2016 (210)

MY OWN MADE EARTH

There is one place I like the best
A place that most people
would never guess

It's here
with my hands
deep in my compost bins
All four of them
large and in a row

Full to the brim with waste and scraps
seaweed, weeds, horse poo
and grounds from my local coffee house

Musty smell of rotting
feeding the worms and the microbes
The damp warmth
and rich dark brown finery
of my own made earth

Then lugged and dug into the garden beds
for the vegetables, for the flowers
for my sheer delighted pleasure

December 2016 (211)

QUITE CERTAIN

I went to sleep
quite certain
of the world and my place

I slept a long dreamy sleep
on perfect pillows
and smooth cotton sheets

My waking was blurry and dazed
and I became alarmed
as I looked out the clear wide window

The world I remembered
I could see through it
right through to the other side
The world that I had known as mine
that had been given to me in a promise

I could no longer help but notice
all that I had so carefully
chosen to ignore

Unnerved and unsure
I could no longer be certain
Quite certain of anything
anymore

December 2016 (212)

THE PERFECT PROMISE

I see you
with your perfect style
your perfect haircut
drinking your almost-perfect coffee

Waiting for your perfect life
Success wrapped in golden titles
secured through well-crafted education
with matching salaries
So you can purchase each and every
perfect parcel of success

I see you
believing these promises
of promotion, prosperity and endless possibilities
Taking the perfect photos on the perfect holiday
Driving your perfect car into this flawless future

I see you
lost in the illusion
pushed from every screen, from every billboard
Finely tuned marketing, perfectly packaged

I see you
endlessly shifting your gaze
from anything that does not fit
this perfect promise

February 2017 (213)

THE STORY THAT'S TOLD

It seems that
everyone wants a big life
Impressive, successful

It seems that
everyone wants
a perfect facebook page
Witty, clever, profound
popular, important

A life judged
by the story that's told
We tick the right boxes
or we fail
We play the game
or we're sidelined

As if we have no quiet joy
no lazy laughter
no slow satisfaction
As if we never struggle
never doubt
never fail

Perpetuating the lie
This simplistic story
of a seemingly
spontaneously and successful life

March 2017 (214)

TUGBOAT

When I was small
I wanted to be
the tugboat skipper
or steer the pilot boat

Be something small that could
push big things around
Out there in the fresh empty air
lots of space and no people

It was a shame I got seasick
And a pity I was a girl

April 2017 (215)

NO MATTER

Having an abusive childhood
a life interrupted
is much like any other chronic condition
We learn to live with it
We learn to manage it
But we never truly recover

No matter how hard we try
no matter how much work we do
no matter who we tell
The stories still remain

No matter who we ask
no matter how many books we read
how many therapists we see
Nothing can save us

No matter how far we run
how many bids for freedom
no matter how many plans we make
There is no escape

No matter how many deals we make
how much we numb or pretend
no matter where we hide
The shadows still chase us

No matter how much noise we make
how much we protest
no matter who we tell
no matter which secrets we keep
The ghosts haunt us

No matter who we become
how much we build
how successful we are
That scared, mistrustful child
can still find us in our quiet

We have to work more
run faster, try harder
to find that place
where most others simply start

There is no tolerable way to explain
Nobody sees

So we hide, we pretend, we struggle
And we fail

April 2017 (216)

TUCKED IN AN ENVELOPE

How do they do it
So self-assured
So decidedly confident
of their place in the world

So definite
that who they are
is good enough
That what they do
is enough

How do they keep
this unfailing belief
in themselves

Is it given out at birth
Do we inherit it from a great-aunt
win it in a raffle
or go buy it somewhere

I thought it might come with age
I might find it in a book
or in the vege garden

Someone might hand it to me
with my morning coffee
or tucked inside the envelope
with my birthday card

Through everything
self-doubt still hangs around
Ready to pounce
whenever I stumble

April 2017 (217)

METICULOUSLY PLANNED

I wish I could believe in a happy future
one that mysteriously does the right thing
That if left alone, unaided
turns out for the best

You toss so much of life into that future
trusting that it will land right side up
knowing there will be time for everything
that there will always be enough

I plan meticulously
protection against doom and chaos
Order must be kept
continuous and conscientious

Just in case life lurches off balance
precarious and unprepared

April 2017 (218)

SIT WITH YOU

I can't help you
All I can do is point to
the prison in your mind

I can't heal you
Just remind you of
your once-trusting heart

I can only sit with you
as you find your way back

Celebrate with you
as you devote yourself
to this moment

August 2017 (219)

STAYING CLOSE ENOUGH

He smells of good things
I knew it
as soon as I stood close enough

Something earthy
a musk that is almost musty
Reminds me of two-day-old
damp mown grass left in rows
on the old school playing field

That smell of the first spring dig
of my waking garden
Summer rain in the forest
the mulch of autumn leaves
smoky winter evening walks

This man
smelling of all things good
Still stays close enough

September 2017 (220)

CHECKING I'M HAPPY

He calls to ask
how my morning had been
that darling husband of mine

I tell him everything I have done
but he just wants to know
that I'd enjoyed myself

So I tell him how well
my tasks have gone
But he just wants to know
that I'm happy

October 2017 (221)

OVERWHELMED

It's everywhere I look
Even the never-really-noticed-before things
they now worry my sleep and disturb my quiet
Those things once taken for granted

The bees' knees and their legs
that carry the pollen
and the other insects too
even the smallest of microbes
are leaving the rich brown earth
And the very soil itself
is being lost to the sea
and the sea rising to meet us
The sea's too warm
for the tiny sea creatures
the big sea creatures being fished into extinction
and the plastic looks like food
they eat it and we eat them
We eat too much
while others are starving

I don't know where it ends

November 2017 (222)

A REAL LIFE BEGINS

Being numb
is to be invisible
Asleep to yourself and any kind of promise
Choosing to feel nothing
is sometimes the best you can do

Being afraid
is better than being numb
But being afraid slowly drains
the life right out of you
until all that is left
is something small
Nobody can see in
It's still better than the nothingness

Feeling angry
is bigger and better than being afraid
But being angry is exhausting and scares the chickens
But at least you feel you are alive
at least something is happening
at least it's a start
Even if it spills out
at least people know you're there

And somewhere after numb
somewhere between the fear and the dread
through the fury and the madness
A real life begins

Courage to move out of the numbness
ignoring the sirens, the alarm bells
the signposts warning of danger

Courage to be scared
Courage to grow big enough
to hold the rage

Courage to forgive

Courage to take your life
back from the past

Claiming
This is now
This is mine

November 2017 (223)

STEALING MY MORNING

It's the morning light that teaches me gratitude
Everything just as I left it
waiting, fresh and familiar

Out of the window, the dewy-new garden
has grown more beautiful through
the resting night into the nourishing light

My lovely's familiar lump in the bed
comforts me that I am still loved
even though he knows me so well

It's the cats who show me that happiness can be found
in a sunny puddle in the middle of the room

All of this before my first sip of my morning coffee
Reminding me that I can still find peace
in this troubled and troubling world

And then into the town
Bombarded by billboards
urgently shouting to acquire, to escape
The huge, defiant and angry cars
The harried people, ears and eyes distracted
willfully absent

It's here that I find it hard to keep despair
from stealing my morning's unruffled ambition

January 2018 (224)

HOW MANY CHANCES

If I have not been enchanted
by one thing
in this long day

Then maybe I am too ungrateful
too full of entitlement
to deserve another

January 2018 (225)

THIS MORNING'S CHORUS

This morning's chorus
was a shambles
Each bird just going for it

No harmonising
no collaboration
no audience awareness
no attention to detail
no Facebook post, no selfies

Just an open-throated and full-bellied
desire to celebrate nothing more
than this day's dawning

My delighted morning ears
stirred my body
my dreamy night brain fell away
and a wee kiss good morning woke my heart

Having taken strict instructions
from the wayward birds
I rolled out of bed
oblivious to anything expected of me

January 2018 (226)

THE STATE OF THE WORLD

If I say these things
you will not like me

If I don't say these things
I will not like myself

Please talk with me
so we can say out loud
those things we don't
want to hear

The more we speak of it
the more we must acknowledge
this is real

Together
we can find the courage
to know
the hard truth

February 2018 (227)

BARE FEET

Feeling something
other than the inside of my shoes
My tender spring feet
touching the sand and the stones

Out on an early evening walk

This dusk is warm and still
a change after
the constant cold sea winds

Summer is promising her annual visit
soon the sea will be ready
for a breathless dip

I'll stay here a little longer
to wait and welcome
her trusted arrival

March 2018 (228)

FULLY IN LOVE

Just because I don't believe in a god
doesn't mean that I never meet with the sacred
Just because I don't give credit to a divining hand
doesn't mean I don't experience what I cannot see

I'm fully in love with beauty and kindness
with courage and joy
My awe at sunrise is no less because
I don't believe it is orchestrated
by someone's god

My appreciation of the bounty of life
stands for me
against a backdrop of chance and disorder
Nothing more than what is real
right here, right now

No need to close my eyes
or sit cross legged

All I need is my garden, the beach, the bush
Any quiet, any beauty, any stillness
will bring me to this deeper conversation
with myself

March 2018 (229)

PROGRESSING

May 2018 - July 2018

A TIME WHEN

I start going to the central library each day and the routine and undisturbed space works a treat. Things start to take shape. I'm making progress, but I'm still on the hunt for a reliable editor.

TOO BIG FOR OUR BRITCHES

Too much of everything
Too big for our britches
as we start to come apart
at the seams

Too much greed
Too much waste
Too little of what we need
Too much of what we don't

Unravelling with every measure

May 2018 (230)

WILBUR WALKING

I walk my neighbour's dog
I don't get Wilbur's fierce loyalty
but I do get his companioned approval

He likes the unleashed beach
where his wild dogness takes over
as he follows every smell
every fast-flying bird
just out of running reach

I trust he knows his limits
He trusts I won't leave him behind

We also walk the nearby bush tracks
Leashed, he has no chance
of chasing the slower birds

I take him for coffee and sometimes a beer
He likes the attention
and in return attends to those
who stop to say a dog-hello

I like to walk my neighbour's dog
Happy to live in a neighbourhood
where we walk each other's dogs
Where we talk to each other
We know each other

May 2018 (231)

GRAB YOUR COAT

Grab your coat
we're going out
Now
Somewhere, there, anywhere

Not when the sun is right
or the wind is light
when the floor is swept
or the inbox cleared

Grab your warmest jacket
this earth can't wait one minute longer
No, we don't have time for me to explain
No, it doesn't matter what shoes you wear

When we are facing into the cold spray
our hands dug deep into warm pockets
We'll witness the sea birds
piloted by wild winds
Feel the small pebbles tremble
as the waves hurtle head-first
arguing incessantly with the shore

June 2018 (232)

JUST NOW

Just now
I finally found enough quiet
to not have to engage
with this urgent and important world

The bone-cold and windless winter-still
drove me inwards
and I was able to hear once more
that sweet and faithful voice

'This small, shy inner-world still wants you'

That was enough
Just enough
To claim my life back
Just now

June 2018 (233)

RUNNING AWAY

We can catch the bus, the train, the plane
as we try and leave our old self behind

But it gets there before us
waiting on the platform
the runway, the doorstep

We can run away
around the corner
to the other side of the world

Our past must still be met
We still need to admit
attend and allow

And then the forgiving

June 2018 (234)

THE PREVAILING QUESTION

It's the right questions
that change the world far more
than the right answers

Grabbing the limelight
answers are as proud as punch
Even when answering the wrong question

Even when answering the right question
self-important answers
believe in themselves perfectly
Forgetting that any answer is just for now

Answers argue, questions wait
Answers spin
questions know their place

Questions endure
Answers come and go

June 2018 (235)

OVER AND OVER

Over and over
the same reply

Have I done well
Am I possibly loved
And still
it's over and over
the same reply

Even when I don't believe the answer
Over and over
it's the same reply

Until my body, the sun, the earth
become the answer
my timetable, my guide
echoing over and over
that same reply

The smile, that look, those words
all tell me the same story
repeating over and over
that same reply

Intimacy comes with each ebb
saturated, yours and mine
and the tides

Over and over
the same reply

June 2018 (236)

SUFFICE

I am ready to abandon the world
Not to die
not unless I have to

But to empty my bags
my mind
my house
of what I thought I wanted

Now
emptied
I'm giving what life
had wanted from me all along

To care for the earth
where I stand
To care for the hearts
given to me in trust

June 2018 (237)

CHOOSING

Choice is a concept
I choose to believe in

It's an idea that helps me
feel less helpless

Ironically however
the less choice
I believe I have
the less I anguish
over my choices

June 2018 (238)

THE MOMENT I NOTICE

I never did find that purpose

By the time I stopped
it didn't matter anymore

The searching ended
the moment I noticed

But I kept walking
the soothing rhythm of my footfall
the steadying horizon

Noticing
Quietly attending

Finding my feet
on this crowded earth

June 2018 (239)

A SIMPLE LIFE

I've worked really hard for a simple life
Saying no is so unfashionable

Going up against the serious significance
the important busyness
of yes

Up to one's ears
in being successful

I thought that saying yes
would bring me a better
more interesting life

Turns out
just made me tired

June 2018 (240)

WHAT REMAINS

I stubbornly spurned
what the world tried to make me
tried to make me believe

As quietly as possible
I didn't want to make a fuss

I almost doubted myself
into a graveyard of conformity
But the grandmothers
soothed and scolded from their crypts
pleading me on

I kicked and rebelled
inner mutiny often ensued
I retreated
but I always returned

I silently screamed and wept myself
inside out

Until I
was all that remained

July 2018 (241)

SOAKED THROUGH

I turned happiness away

I tried to explain
about the problems of the world
my own troubles
the angst and the anguish

Happiness persisted
Showing up everywhere
Never listening to a word

Until my resolve it broke
and happiness flooded through
soaking everything

July 2018 (242)

MY ONLY PROMISE

I am willing
That is my only promise

The only promise to you
the only promise to life

This oath to myself

Less resistance
more willingness
That is my only promise

July 2018 (243

ENDLESS HOURS

I remember those times
the corner shop where I bought my milkshakes
roaming the neighbourhood
nobody watching
nobody needing to

Ant trails and summer plums
endless hours playing until after dusk
just enough light to find our way home

Even though my childhood home was hard
it was still full of stretchy time

Now
the hours merge
the days collapse into one another
Time spreads like butter on hot toast
and before I know it
breakfast is done

July 2018 (244)

NATURE'S LISTENING IN

She lives downstream
from every greedy industry

She lives in the middle
of each mindless rubbish dump

She lives in the sea creatures'
plastic-filled bellies
hungry too

She drinks from the poisoned rivers
and roams the same lost
and treeless landscapes

She lines our rubbish bins

She knows our mischief
She hears our conversations
Eavesdrops on every deal
that takes her to market to be sold

Outvoted by big business and progress
Out marketed by privilege and power

But on the last vote
the laws of nature win
No matter what the courts
the spreadsheets or the boards decide

In the end
Nature has the final say

July 2018 (245)

WILDS OF THE LOST

When I take care of the wee hurt me
she slowly wanders back up the long path
emerging from the wilds of the lost

She is brave
to be both
expectant and afraid

I never quite know what to do

But I will not leave her
Not again
Not like everyone else
Not again
Not like that

July 2018 (246)

UNCONCERNED

I think the trees are happy with their view
taking their growing-time
Arching sideways with the steady wind
Satisfied with their place in the forest
the orchard, or at the bottom of my garden

The river changes course
after long and fierce consultation
with the droughts and the storms

The weeds, the flower buds, my vegetables
grow together and apart
win their place or lose

Seeds move on the breeze
the insides of birds
on the edge of my skirt

Or not

July 2018 (247)

LOVE AFFAIR

Nature and I have been holding hands
whispering sweet sounds
being gracious
for a long time now

Dressing in linen shirts
tending my garden
walking on the beaches
These aren't enough any more
The time for courting is over

I need to find my way back to the earth
I want deep kisses and feral love-making
I want more

Having been jilted and forsaken before
Nature is demanding total commitment
No more flirting around the edges

To prove myself by placing her
above all my other loves
To care for her with all my heart
and in all my living

Fair enough I say
Fair enough

July 2018 (248)

FINDING THE TREASURES

Those with the definite answers
the ones who think they know
They stand on the lecterns
stand for Parliament
they put their names to the opinion pieces
write the contracts
dictate the terms

Those with more and many questions
they are making music
giving comfort
Reticent, they curiously wander
the great halls of beauty
Finding treasures

July 2018 (249)

ON WAKING

I went to sleep quite safe in my dreamy bed
trusting in an innocent and noble sleep
but awoke to a tangled mess

Right between my belly and my heart
wet rags of doubt
tossed about
Tied into clumps of foreboding
Touchy bundles of misgivings

Cheated of a replenishing sleep
I awoke diminished
In my deep sleepy rest
my defences had weakened
the old stories had swarmed in

I so needed the beauty of that morning
to help me rearrange
myself back into the present

To choose again
the goodness of my grown-up life

July 2018 (250)

SAVED

But nobody, nothing saved me

I had to plan and execute
the whole manoeuvre
by myself
It was clumsy and inefficient

But I got away, anyway

I did leave it till the very last minute
still hoping for a piece-of-cake escape

Willing rescuers aren't as common
as the storybooks proclaim

At large
Released
Unhinged perhaps

But free

July 2018 (251)

RANSACKED

What can I do with this small
almost-finished life

What can I do now, next
As I feel the grief
of the natural world
slipping through our fingers
As we grasp
for the next and the next
and still our hands and hearts
are left empty

And again, tomorrow
What can I do
with this one small
almost finished life

July 2018 (252)

SITTING ON THE DOORSTEP

It is useless
to go out in search of love
if on return
all the windows and doors
are still bolted shut

Stay home and do the work
until the windows and doors
swing freely on their hinges

Clear the garden path
make some tea
sit on the doorstep
and wait

July 2018 (253)

WADING THROUGH MUD

August 2018 – July 2019

A TIME WHEN

I do some full-on therapy about my childhood abuse. It's good stuff, but in the process my brain falls out. Around the same time the library closes, and other things happen that need my attention. Spend a lot of time waiting for editors and it feels like wading through mud.

DOING NO HARM

So few places left
to sit with nature
doing no harm

Thumping waves
punching angrily at the shore

Tender tides
kissing the sand

A rhythmic swell
telling tidal time's ancient story

I long to sit here a little longer
doing no harm

November 2018 (254)

RIVER TALK

Rivers change colour with the weather, with the seasons
Rivers bite when they are cold
rouse us when we are hot and sluggish

Rivers smell good

River music
changes its song with the rain
and plays duets with the summer swimmers

Rivers talk
they console and reassure
they answer back
Rivers tell their stories
to our children and our grandchildren
They teach us

Rivers carry life

Rivers shouldn't disappear
Rivers shouldn't get sick from abuse
Rivers shouldn't die
from neglect

December 2018 (255)

BEING LOST

I'm in and out of that door
The one leading into the world

Sitting on the doorstep
legs pulled up
leaning back against the door frame
I am neither in nor out

Scared of losing myself in here
Those old voices inside my head
still giving bad advice
The sickness in the pit of my belly
already ready to spread
Dreading those nauseating feeling
Scared of crumbling in on top of myself
Buried alive

Scared of out there too
Swamped
Never sure which way to go
Swept away
Vanishing into the crowding
Unbalanced by the constant and continual bustle
Clamouring

I sit in the doorframe
Scared of being lost in here
Scared of being lost out there

December 2018 (256)

QUIET NOW

I have no problem
with silence

Sometimes I wish the whole world
would shut-up

Including me

March 2019 (257)

TALKING ABOUT CLIMATE

If I say these things
you will not like me

If I don't say these things
I will not like myself

April 2019 (258)

HARDLY EVER

There used to be dead insects stuck
on the windscreen whenever
we drove a longish way, or at night
small green bottles of 'Bar's Bugs' windscreen cleaner
tucked away in the glove box

Now
not so much
Now
hardly at all

We have killed them
with our chemicals and insecticides
And all the land, their homes, their food is
ordered and tidy
Used up

The garden once hummed all summer long
the air shimmering and alive

Small mounds on the windowsills
of dead and dying bugs
caught on the inside of the glass

Not now
not so much
hardly at all
if ever

July 2019 (259)

OUT INTO THE WORLD

March 2020 – June 2021

A TIME WHEN

I pull back from my business, thanks to a supportive husband. I keep plugging away, and in the end my brain finds me again. I finally find the perfect editor. Turns out to be my husband and we work well together.

I finally get these books out into the world. I'm delighted, relieved and satisfied.

ACKNOWLEDGEMENTS

Most importantly to my husband Peter, for giving me the space and encouragement to fulfill my lifetime dream of being a writer. Even though it has taken way longer than he -and I - thought.

To my children who always believe in me, even when I don't.

To my close friends, for reading through the many drafts and giving such useful feedback.

Again to Peter for his honest and insightful editing.

To all my friends and clients. Thanks for the support, the teaching, the endless rants, and the love and laughs.

ABOUT THE AUTHOR

Jane lives in Wellington, New Zealand with her husband Peter. She spends her days tending her garden, walking her dog, and writing. She still sometimes works as a mediator, facilitator, and communications coach and presenter.

She has written two other books: *Follow Yourself Home* and *In Your Smallest Pocket*.

For more information and for book purchases, go to her website: www.wordremedies.co.nz

Alternatively, you can purchase ebooks and physical books directly from Amazon, or other similar platforms.

INDEX OF REMEDY TITLES

and first lines

D

E

F

G

H

I

J

K

L

M

N

O

P

Q

R

S

T

Y

Made in United States
North Haven, CT
10 November 2026

22096549R00192